Vegan

Low Carb Diet Guide for Beginners with Easy and Quick for Weight loss

(Over 50 Easy and Healthy Recipes to Get Started)

Joe Beam

Published by Robert Satterfield Publishing House

© **Joe Beam**

All Rights Reserved

Vegan Diet: Low Carb Diet Guide for Beginners with Easy and Quick for Weight loss (Over 50 Easy and Healthy Recipes to Get Started)

ISBN 978-1-989787-04-5

All rights reserved. No part of this guide may be reproduced in any form without permission in writing from the publisher except in the case of brief quotations embodied in critical articles or reviews.

Legal & Disclaimer

The information contained in this book is not designed to replace or take the place of any form of medicine or professional medical advice. The information in this book has been provided for educational and entertainment purposes only.

The information contained in this book has been compiled from sources deemed reliable, and it is accurate to the best of the Author's knowledge; however, the Author cannot guarantee its accuracy and validity and cannot be held liable for any errors or omissions. Changes are periodically made to this book. You must consult your doctor or get professional medical advice before using any of the suggested remedies, techniques, or information in this book.

TABLE OF CONTENT

Part 1 1

Introduction... 2

WHY ADOPT A VEGAN DIET 4
A HEALTHY VEGAN EATING HABIT 15

Vegan Diet Recipes 23

Roasted Tofu With Peanuts.. 23

Mushroom Teriyaki 24

Roasted Cauliflower Bites... 26

Guacamole With Tomatoes 27

Baked Onion Bhajis... 28

Breakfast 30

Tofu Scrambled With Roasted Tomatoes........................... 30

Pumpkin Muffins 32

Cashew Cream And Fruit Parfait 35

Vegan French Toast 36

Maple-Nut Granola... 37

Avocado Quinoa Bowl 39

Three-Bean Salad 40

Spiralized Asian Quinoa Salad With Peanut Dressing......... 42

Chickpea Salad... 44

Sweet Potato And Beans 45

- Sesame Noodles 46
- Vegetable Soup 48
- Bean And Rice Soup... 49
- Snacks.. 51
- Chickpea Wraps... 52
- Veggie Chilli 54
- Apple Green Smoothie 54
- Chilled Cantaloupe Soup 55
- Mint Chocolate Smoothie 56
- Fruit Tart With Caramel Almond Filling........................... 57
- Desserts... 58
- Chocolate Raspberry Smoothie 59
- Piña Colada Smoothie 59
- Banana Berry Smoothie.. 60
- Peanut Butter S'moreos 61
- Peanut Butter Fudge 62
- 30. Vegan Chocolate Milkshake 63
- Conclusion 64
- Part 2 65
- Introduction.. 66
- Chalupas 68
- Ron's Best Guacamole.. 69

- Jicama Con Limon Y Chile 70
- Sopa De Nopal (Cactus Soup) 71
- Tequila Avocado Soup 72
- Textured Vegetable Protein Mole Enchiladas 73
- Red Mole Sauce (Makes 2 Cups) 75
- Mexican Rice With Vegetables 76
- Stuffed Cabbage In Chipotle Sauce 77
- Chiles Rellenos... 79
- Chiles Rellenos Stuffed With Brown Rice 81
- Salsa Mexicana 83
- Banana Flambé 84
- Salsa Chipotle 85
- Fennel A La Grecque... 86
- Caramelised Fennel 88
- Grilled Asparagus With Blood Oranges And Tapenade Toast 89
- Moroccan Chickpeas 91
- Eggplant, Tomato And Onion Gratin 93
- Bean Ragout With Potato Gnocchi...................................... 94
- Potato, Morel And Onion Fricassee.................................... 96
- Sichuan Kung Pao 'Chicken'.. 98
- Stir-Fried Tofu With Leeks 100

- Vegetarian Stir Fry 'Oyster' Sauce ... 101
- Sichuan 'Beef' And Broccoli ... 102
- Red Pepper Tofu ... 104
- Mapo Doufu ... 106
- Hunan Hot And Sour Vegetarian "Duck" ... 108
- Steamed Tofu With Spicy Bean Paste Sauce ... 110
- Hunan Style "Duck" Curry ... 112
- Hunan Tofu With Fresh Garlic ... 114
- Chinese-Style Chili Green Beans ... 116
- Chinese-Style Zucchini With Ginger ... 118
- Sichuan Spicy Tangerine 'Chicken' ... 119
- Dan Dan Noodles ... 121
- Gluten Dough ... 123
- Buddha's "Chicken" ... 125
- Chinese Style "Beefy" Seitan ... 127
- Asparagus Beef With Black Bean Sauce ... 130
- Onion-Fragrant Red Lentils ... 132
- Tart Red Lentils ... 134
- Green Split Peas In Zesty Mustard Sauce ... 136
- Down Home Chick Pea Stew ... 138
- Festive Chickpeas With Coconut And Whole Spices ... 140
- Fiery Potatoes ... 142

- Spicy Home Fries 144
- Potatoes Braised In Rich Tart Sauce 146
- Potato Skin Fry 148
- Rich Roasted Eggplant 150
- Butternut Squash In Mustard Sauce.................................. 152
- Cabbage Potato Extravaganza.. 154
- Steamed Spicy Cauliflower 156
- Cauliflower And Potatoes In Roasted Red Chilli Sauce..... 157
- Spicy Stuffed Tomatoes... 161
- Pureed Greens With Chilli And Coconut Over Rice 163
- Vegetable Pullao.. 165
- Puffed Bread.. 168
- Coconut Scented Rice Pudding... 170
- Poppy Seed Sauce 171
- Crisp Fried Eggplant.. 173
- Sweet And Tart Pumpkin.. 174
- Peanut Topped Greens... 176
- Lime Splashed Butternut Squash Over Rice 178
- Coconut And Cilantro Chutney... 179
- Hot And Spicy Bean Curd Burritos..................................... 180
- Biker Beerittos... 182
- Put Tortilla On A Plate. 183

Mean Black Bean Soup	185
Angel Pasta	187
Hot Nutty Noodles	190
Smoky Bean Curd Stir Fry	192
Hot Garbanzo Beans With Sun Dried	195
Masala Potatoes	196
Mexicorn	198
Hot Nutty Butternut	199
Killer Curry	204
Polka Pepper Pasta	206
Loco Lo Mien	208
Red Hot Red Pepper Salsa	211
About The Author	213

Part 1

Introduction

This book contains proven steps and strategies on how to maintain a healthy, high protein diet for vegans, with 30 quick and easy recipes.

For those of us who have been reading and listening to news regarding health and diet, your attention must have been drawn to the contentious issues of whether or not to consume animal products. The debate rages from how much to consume, what to avoid, what to take in moderation and it seems to go on and on. Is it not tiring, to believe in one thing and be led to another supposed truth shortly afterwards? If you want to learn everything about the vegan diet, then this book is what you need.

This book is the key to all there is to know about the vegan diet. You will learn what veganism is all about, the different types of vegans there are, the benefits of adopting a vegan diet as well as some tasty recipes that you could try at home.

Join me in this lovely adventure of a healthy lifestyle.

Thanks again for downloading this book, I hope you enjoy it!

Vegan Diet vs. Meat Diet

Every other day, there seems to be a new diet that has been developed. However, most of us are aware of the two variations, the "vegetarian diet", and the "meat diet" which will serve as the baseline of our discussion.

A meat diet allows you to eat animal products as well as a variety of vegetables. Restrictions come in with the vegetarian diet, which is free from meat, poultry, and fish. However, as a vegetarian, you can eat some animal products. Lacto-vegetarians can consume dairy products while lacto-ovo-vegetarians can consume both dairy products and eggs.

Vegans are a lot similar to vegetarians but not only do they refrain from the use of animal products but their byproducts too.

This means that as a vegan, you should not consume dairy products, eggs and the non-consumables too like silk, leather, soap, wool cosmetics, and other products that are derived from animals. Therefore, instead of joining the debate of what quantity of animal products is healthy, vegans avoid it all together and concentrate on the other healthy vegan products.

So, what exactly do you stand to benefit from being a vegan? Let us find out.

Why Adopt A Vegan Diet

There are many advantages of being a vegan ranging from being protective of animal rights to environmental concerns and our well-being. Since health matters concern us most, my inclination is to outline to you the health benefits of following a vegan lifestyle.

It lowers LDL (bad) cholesterol levels

You have definitely come across cholesterol especially when reading about the effects of diet to your health.

Cholesterol is a waxy substance found in all cells. The scientists term it as a friend as well as a foe; a friend because the body needs it to make hormones and other substances needed for digestion. We normally get cholesterol from the food we eat and it is transported in the form of lipids. So when does cholesterol become a foe? When the levels of cholesterol are high in the body, they are deposited in the inner linings of your blood vessels, which can later cause serious complications, as we will come to see later.

You must be wondering what cholesterol has to do with a vegan diet. High cholesterol levels have been attributed to an unhealthy diet of meat, poultry, and dairy products. Actually, to cut down on your cholesterol level, you need to restrict your consumption of animal products. As a vegan, you will not be eating animal products and this will greatly reduce your bad cholesterol levels. The good news is that you will still be getting the amount of cholesterol your body needs since your liver produces enough of the needed cholesterol to carry out the necessary body functions.

Reduces risk of heart diseases

Studies conducted among populations of people on meat and vegan diets have shown that most of the people affected by heart diseases and hypertension come from those who eat animal products. This can be attributed to the fact that animal products have a high cholesterol level. So how does high cholesterol level lead to hypertension and heart diseases? Gradual deposition of cholesterol in the blood vessels leads to narrowing of the lumen. Take an example of a pipe, if you keep on depositing large debris and fat in your sink, it keeps on collecting at the base of the pipe. With time, they solidify and make the lumen of the pump narrower. If you had to pass water through the pipe, then you would have to use much more force than if the lumen was larger.

That is the same effect that the blood vessels have against the heart. The heart has to work extra hard to push blood against resistance from the blood vessels. This later leads to the heart muscles enlarging and finally failing to perform their work efficiently.

The narrowing blood vessels also cause a rise in the blood pressure hence hypertension sets in. The clogging of the vessels can impede proper flow of blood especially in the small vessels supplying the heart known as the coronary heart vessels. This leads to coronary artery diseases a precursor for a heart attack.

Taking a vegan diet protects you from these killer diseases, as it is free from cholesterol.

Reduces the risk of obesity

Obesity has been cited as a contributory factor to many diseases both physical and emotional. You will be surprised to find out that it isn't prevalent among the vegan population. This is because the vegan diet has high fiber content and adequate levels of protein unlike a diet composed of animal products. This is not to say that animal products do not have adequate protein. On the contrary, they have more than enough. However, you do not only get protein but unhealthy fats too. Fats are an essential component of the diet, but can either be healthy or unhealthy.

There are two types of harmful dietary fat namely saturated fats and the trans-fats. Animal products like full fat dairy products, red meat, and poultry are the sources of saturated fats. On the other hand, plants are the main sources of healthy fats. These are the poly-unsaturated fats, which are from plant based oils and foods, and the omega 3 fats from the nuts and seeds of the vegan diet.

Intake of harmful fats results in a high cholesterol level subjecting you to the above dangers and the risk of being obese. The potential dangers of being obese are clear to most of us and going vegan is of way of avoiding the predisposing factors.

Reduces chances of suffering from cancer

Studies have shown that diet also has an effect on some types of cancer. Colorectal cancer has been associated with a diet high in processed foods and red meat. Studies have also shown that the incidence of this type of cancer among vegans is lower than those who consume animal products. In addition to vegans avoiding meat, it has been noted that vegans have a lower secondary bile acids in feces. This means that they are less likely to have infrequent bowel movements, which also serves as a protective factor.

The other type of cancer that is less prevalent among vegans is breast cancer. This may come as a shock because breast cancer has been associated with hormonal factors especially estrogen. Studies show that there is known difference of estrogen levels in both vegans and those who consume animal products. However, the insulin growth factor 1 has also been cited to increase the risks of breast cancer. Vegans have been shown to have lower levels of the insulin growth factor 1; thus, lowering the risks of getting breast cancer. The same principle is true for prostate cancer.

The above mentioned are some of the few health advantages of adopting a vegan diet. However, in order to enjoy the mentioned benefits, it is important to ensure that you do not have nutritional deficiencies. Therefore, in the following chapter, we will look at important things that you should note when going vegan.

Important Things To Note About A Vegan Diet

Most of us are aware of what a healthy diet is composed of, the nutrients that the body needs which are carbohydrates, proteins, vitamins, minerals, and fats. For most of us that have been brought up in families that are not vegan, our view of a balanced diet is somewhat distorted and we believe that the only way for our diet to be balanced is to have grains as carbohydrates, animal products as proteins, vegetables and fruits as our main source of vitamins. Thus, it becomes a little tricky to balance the vegan plate and most of the time, we fail to take enough of specific nutrients and this leads to nutritional deficiencies, which is what you don't want. Thus, in this section, we will look at some nutrients that most vegans are likely not to have adequate of and how to ensure you eat enough of these nutrients.

Proteins

Proteins are essential for growth and are referred to as the body building foods. Animal products and byproducts might be a good source of protein but not the sole source. As a vegan, your source of proteins will be from:

- Legumes; different types of peas, beans, and lentils
- Soy and soy products
- Different types of nuts (hazelnuts, almonds, peanuts) and seeds (sesame, sunflower)

Iron

Iron is a necessary component of hemoglobin, which is a component of red blood cells. The function of hemoglobin is to circulate oxygen from the lungs to the other parts of the body. If you lack iron, you are likely to suffer from a condition known as iron deficiency anemia where the hemoglobin level is too low to sustain the normal processes of the body. Both vegetables and animal products are rich in iron. The only difference is that iron from the animal products is readily absorbed unlike iron from vegetables. This may come as a disadvantage to vegans but one that can easily be overcome. As a vegan, focus on eating meals that either contain iron or those that have been fortified with iron. Some of the examples are:

- Beans, peas and lentils
- Nuts
- Vegetables
- Grain products that have been fortified with iron
- Prunes and apricots

In addition to this, take iron supplements and make sure you take it with citrus juice or anything rich in vitamin C, which helps in the absorption of iron.

Calcium

Most of us know milk is important since it is rich in calcium. The body uses most of the calcium in ensuring we have healthy bones and teeth. It is also important for ensuring skeletal stability. In addition, it plays a vital role in blood clotting, cell signaling, nerve function, and muscle contraction. So, what is your alternative source of calcium? Below are some suitable sources of calcium:

- Fruits like figs and fortified orange juice
- Vegetables like collard greens, turnip greens, okra and Bok Choy
- Sesame butter
- Blackstrap molasses

If the above is not readily available, you can use calcium supplements.

Vitamin B12

Vitamin B12 is an important component in protein metabolism. Just like iron, the body readily absorbs vitamin B12 from animal sources rather than plant sources. It is also important for healthy skin, hair, eyes, and even liver. It also ensures proper functioning of the nervous system. Some sources of vitamin B12 include:

- Fortified beverages; soy, almond and rice beverages
- Red star nutritional yeast

- Vitamin B12 supplements; daily at 10 micrograms or weekly at 2000 micrograms

Omega 3 fats

Omega 3 fatty acids are considered as essential fats needed by the body. They are an important part of cell membrane and ensure proper functioning of cell receptors. They also ensure efficiency in other hormonal functions in the body like the contraction and relaxation of blood vessels, blood clotting, and play a major role in inflammation. Unfortunately, the body is unable to manufacture omega 3 fatty acids and must obtain them from food. Some good sources of omega 3 fatty acids include;

- Nuts especially walnuts
- Seeds; flax seeds and flax seed oils
- Leafy vegetables

A Healthy Vegan Eating habit

Having ensured that you have included the above in your diet, maintaining a healthy vegan-eating pattern becomes easier. To make sure that you do this right, below are the recommended servings of each food group in a vegan diet.

Maintain 2 ½ cups of vegetables a day

Dark green – 1 ½ cups a day

Legumes (beans and peas) – 3 cups a week

Starchy vegetables – 3 cups a week

Fruits – 2 cups a day

Maintain 6 ½ ounces of grains a day

Whole grains – more than 3 ½ ounces a day

Refined grains – less than 3 ounces a day

Maintain 3 ½ ounces protein a day

Nuts, soy products, and seeds – 14 ounces a week

Vegetable oils 27 grams a day

A Healthy Way Of Easily Adopting To The Vegan Diet

The challenge of getting into any new thing is not having an idea of it and doing it the wrong way. The unfortunate thing with a diet is you are bound to make mistakes that can be detrimental to your health. As you get into the vegan way of life, I would like you to be able to reap 100% of the benefits. You will only achieve this if you do not feel miserable about the diet and are taking in the right combination of nutrients. Here are some tips to help you as you adopt a vegan lifestyle:

Educate yourself

This has been the purpose of the book all along, to get you to know the basics of a vegan diet. You will not be able to adopt a healthy vegan lifestyle if you do not understand the difficulties, the benefits, and the challenges of the diet. Furthermore, if you have a knowledge deficit of the above, it becomes easier for you to be derailed and lose focus.

We also do not want to endanger you by letting you experience nutritional deficiencies. More reasons why you have to be clear on planning your plate, reading the nutritional labels, and not overindulging in any specific meal while leaving out another nutritious one. Some tips of going through this are;

Learning how to read labels: this might be the only way to sort out vegan friendly and non-vegan friendly foods. As discussed earlier, being vegan is a little more complicated that simply being a vegetarian.

You also have to know the difference between natural, processed, and organic foods. Organic foods are those that are grown without the use of fertilizers, additional growth hormones, or antibiotics. Natural foods do not require any special listings like those of organic foods while the processed foods are those that are loaded with preservatives, dyes, sweeteners and all other imitations that you can think of.

Learn of the different substitutes for dairy products, honey, and butter: You can substitute milk with soymilk. You can also substitute butter with vegetable-based butter. Ground flax seed is a good substitute for eggs. For the recipes that usually need you to add honey, you can use agave syrup/nectar or maple syrup instead. You can also use tofu in place of cheese. Tofu can be used in many foods either baked or fried. When made with vegetables it resembles scrambled eggs.

Clearing out your kitchen

Clearing out your kitchen of animal products and byproducts is important to making the transition to a vegan lifestyle. It is not easy to go through with it overnight. You need to plan, set and clarify your goals and start weaning off animals products. You could start with meat products by first eliminating red meat followed by white meat. This leaves you at the vegetarian stage, which is a little easier to cope. After that, eliminate the dairy products and finally the poultry e.g. eggs. As you go through with eliminations of these products from the diet purchase vegan foods. We will talk more about what to buy later on.

Create a meal plan; start with the basics of what you know

Make a grocery list and later go shopping

Buy healthy vegan friendly foods

As you clean out your kitchen of animal products and by products, you need to fill the kitchen with vegan diet foods. You should already have educated yourself on the diet and laid a plan on how to execute it. The next thing is to purchase vegan foods. Buy vegetables, legumes, fruits, nuts, and seeds not forgetting healthy vegetable cooking oils. Spice it up a little with the different types of herbs and condiments like mustard, tahini, tamari, stevia, balsamic and apple cider vinegar sand others that you know, as you open up to a new world. Do not forget to get healthy grains like quinoa. You may need to have alternatives during this transition period; getting things like unsweetened almond milk in place of dairy would be a good idea. You could use it with your breakfast cereals, hemp, chia, or walnuts.

Focus on the basic

You will realize that there are not many changes after withdrawal of animal products and you could start from where you are. I term this as focusing on the basic. A good example would be your breakfast; you may probably be used to taking cereals and dairy milk. Having eliminated the dairy milk and replaced it with almond milk you are good to go. Actually, you could spice this up a little by adding in some cinnamon, chopped fruit and some coconut yoghurt. There are several soups that I will later share with you for your lunch, meanwhile rice and some legumes will do just fine. You also have a variety of starchy vegetables like potatoes. Top it up with vegetables most of which you are already familiar with. Nuts and seeds will make good snacks.

Find tasty recipes

To ensure you don't get bored with the same meals over and over again, familiarize yourself with new ways of preparing your food. It is critical to have variety in your meals and thanks to this book, you will learn many meals that you can prepare. Pick out favorites and keep on learning new ones.

Eat whole foods

You have to make cooking your friend and avoid buying processed foods. The reason I would not advise on eating out is because you cannot be 100% sure of the ingredients and you might be introduced to unhealthy components that you are trying to avoid in the first place. Go for shopping and pick out healthy whole foods. Once you have a meal plan, it is easy to prepare the food that you need for the day. If you work, you could pack some and carry it in a lunch box so that you do not have to go hungry or worse, eat the unhealthy processed meals.

Factor in the supplements

With the vegan diet, you must be ready to take supplements faithfully. We already discussed the nutrients that are not readily absorbed from plants, which include vitamin B12 and iron. Make a point of taking the recommended amount of supplements as recommended. Also, eat the food that has been fortified with them too as discussed. You will find many food products fortified with the minerals. You must be keen in reading the nutritional labels in order to ensure you eat healthy foods.

Vegan Diet Recipes

Appetizers

Roasted tofu with peanuts
Yields: 1 cup
Ingredients
1 ½ tablespoons chili oil

1 ounce fried peanuts

3 celery stalks

3 ½ ounces smoked firm tofu

Salt, to taste

Pinch of sugar

Directions

1. Cut the tofu into 3/8-inch cubes and then de-string the celery, cut lengthways into ½ inch strips then into smaller pieces like the tofu.

2. Boil water in a pot, add the celery, and blanch for about 1 minute; ensure the celery is still crunchy.

3. Transfer the celery to a colander and cool under running cold water, and shake dry.

4. Combine all ingredients in a medium bowl, mix and serve.

Mushroom Teriyaki

Serves 4-6

Ingredients

16 ounces fresh mushrooms

Freshly ground pepper to taste

Fresh herbs you like for garnish

Teriyaki Sauce

1 teaspoon grated ginger

1-2 cloves minced garlic

1 tablespoon rice vinegar

2 teaspoons granulated sugar

1 tablespoon dark sesame oil

2 tablespoons white wine

2 tablespoons reduced-sodium soy sauce

Directions

1. Combine all the ingredients for the sauce in a small container and stir; set aside.

2. Wipe the mushrooms clean then mix them with just enough water in a pan to keep the bottom moist.

3. Cover and cook over medium high heat for about 5 minutes or until the mushrooms just start to soften.

4. Pour out the liquid from the pan and add in the sauce you made. Increase the heat and cook until the sauce forms a

glaze on mushrooms; season salt and pepper.

5. Transfer to a platter and garnish with herbs.

Roasted cauliflower bites
Serves 6

Ingredients

½ teaspoon garlic powder

½ teaspoon smoked paprika

½ teaspoon ground cumin

½ teaspoon salt

1 teaspoon chili powder

1 head cauliflower

Directions

1. Preheat the oven to 400 degrees F.

2. Use parchment paper to line a baking sheet.

3. Cut the cauliflower into florets, rinse under running water, and shake off the

excess water. Spread the florets on a baking sheet.

4. Mix all seasonings in a bowl, sprinkle on the cauliflower ensuring you turn the florets so that all sides are seasoned.

5. Bake in the oven for 15 minutes, turn the florets, and bake for 15 more minutes.

6. Remove and serve with any dipping sauce you like.

Guacamole with tomatoes
Serves 4

Ingredients

3 avocados, peeled, stones removed and mashed

1 pinch ground cayenne pepper

1 clove garlic, minced

2 plum tomatoes, diced

1 small handful chopped fresh coriander

½ diced onion

1 teaspoon salt

1 lime, juiced

Directions

1. Mix together avocados, salt and lime juice. Add in the tomatoes, coriander and onion and mix. Stir in cayenne pepper and refrigerate for around 1 hour for best flavor.

2. Serve with corn bread cubes or some crackers.

Baked onion bhajis

Makes 8 bhajis

Ingredients

For the bhaji mix

1 tablespoon tomato puree

Extra virgin olive oil, as needed

½ teaspoon ground coriander

½ teaspoon ground cumin

1 pinch salt

5 tablespoons chickpea flour

5 small onions, sliced 5mm thick

Water, as needed

Spices for the pan

¼ teaspoon chili powder

¼ teaspoon ground ginger

¼ teaspoon ground cumin

½ teaspoon ground coriander

½ teaspoon ground turmeric

Directions

1. Preheat the oven to 200 degrees Celsius.

2. Use parchment paper to line a baking tray.

3. Cook the onions in a pan with oil for about 6-8 minutes or until translucent.

4. Add in the chili powder and mix, and then add coriander, ginger, cumin, and turmeric and stir; remove from the heat.

5. Put the chickpea flour, cumin, coriander, and salt in a bowl and mix well. Add tomato puree and onions into the bowl and mix. You can add in a little water to achieve the right consistency; the mixture should be wet but not sloppy.

6. Drizzle oil onto the prepared baking tray, put 2 tablespoons of onion mix on each try for every bhaji, and flatten using the back of a spoon.

7. Bake for about 25 minutes, drizzle some oil on top and bake for about 25 more minutes; serve hot and enjoy.

Breakfast

Tofu scrambled with roasted tomatoes
Serves 4

Ingredients

4 tomatoes

1 tablespoon red wine vinegar

2 tablespoons olive oil, divided

1 tablespoon brown sugar

2 teaspoons dried mixed herbs

¼ tablespoon freshly ground black pepper

¼ tablespoon kosher salt

2 teaspoons ground turmeric

2 teaspoons garlic powder

2 (14-ounces) packages extra firm dried tofu, drained

2 zucchini, diced

1 yellow onion diced

1 red bell pepper, diced

½ cup nutritional yeast

8 ounces button mushrooms, sliced

Directions

1. Preheat the oven to 400 degrees F.

2. Cut the tomatoes into quarters then cut each quarter into half crosswise.

3. Toss the tomatoes, a tablespoon of olive oil, vinegar, pepper and salt in a medium bowl and transfer to a baking sheet.

4. Bake for 25-30 minutes until soft and caramelized.

5. Combine garlic powder, dried herbs, and turmeric in another medium mixing bowl.

6. Crumble the tofu into the same bowl, mix then set aside.

7. Heat a large skillet over medium heat. Add the remaining tablespoon of oil and cook the onion for 4 minutes until soft.

8. Add mushrooms, bell pepper and zucchini, and cook for 5 minutes until tender.

9. Add the nutritional yeast and tofu and cook for 4 minutes until heated through.

10. Serve with roasted tomatoes.

Pumpkin muffins

Makes 12 muffins

Ingredients

Wet ingredients

1 cup unsweetened pumpkin puree

1 tablespoon chia seeds

3 tablespoons pure maple syrup

¼ cup blackstrap molasses

1/3 cup grape seed oil or melted coconut oil

½ cups packed brown sugar

3 tablespoons water

Dry ingredients

1 tablespoon pumpkin pie spice

1 2/3 cups whole grain spelt flour

1 teaspoon baking soda

½ teaspoon fine sea salt

1 teaspoon baking powder

Heaping ½ cup toasted chopped walnuts.

Directions

1. Preheat the oven to 350 degrees F.

2. Line the muffin pans with paper liners and whisk the chia seeds and water in a medium bowl.

3. Set it aside for a few minutes to thicken.

4. Mix the dry ingredients in a large bowl.

5. Add the wet ingredients to the chia mixture and whisk until smooth

6. Add the wet mixture into the large bowl with dry ingredients and stir until just combined (ensure that no patches of flour remain but do not over-mix the batter); the batter will be quite thick.

7. Stir in the chopped walnuts and reserve some for garnish.

8. Divide the batter between the 12 muffin liners. Ensure they are ¾ full.

9. Add the reserved walnuts on the top and push down gently.

10. Bake the muffins for 20-24 muffins; use a toothpick to test, it should come out clean

11. Cool the muffins in a pan for 5-10 minutes and then transfer them onto a cooling rack until cool.

12. Serve with almond milk

Tips

- To make the pumpkin puree less grainy, throw it into a food processor and blend until smooth
- If using coconut oil, all the other ingredients should be at room temperature
- You can use all- purpose flour as an alternative

Cashew cream and fruit parfait

Serves 4

Ingredients

1 cup raw cashews

1 tablespoon maple syrup

¼ cup cold water

¼ teaspoon vanilla extract

1 teaspoon lemon zest

Pinch fine sea salt

2 cups fresh fruits of your choice

Directions

1. Place the cashews in a bowl and cover with warm water.

2. Let it sit overnight or for a minimum of 6 hours.

3. Drain the cashews and place in a blender with water, maple syrup, lemon zest and salt and blend until smooth.

4. Layer the fresh fruit, 2 heaping tablespoons cashew cream, more fruit, then 2 more tablespoons of cashew cream then the rest of the fruits in a parfait glass. Serve.

Vegan French toast

Serves 2-3

Ingredients

6 slices ciabatta bread, sliced about ¾ inch thick

¼ teaspoon freshly ground nutmeg

1 teaspoon cinnamon

1 tablespoon nutritional yeast

2 tablespoon millet flour

1 tablespoon maple syrup, plus more for serving

1 cup almond milk

Coconut oil, for the pan

Pinch of salt

Toppings

Powdered sugar

Maple syrup

Vegan butter

Fresh fruit

Directions

1. Whisk together flour, salt, nutmeg, cinnamon, nutritional yeast and maple syrup in a small bowl.

2. Put the bread in a shallow dish then pour the above mixture over the bread. Flip the bread to ensue both sides are coated evenly with the mixture.

3. Heat some coconut oil in a skillet over medium heat. Once the pan is hot, putt eh bread slices and cook each side for a few minutes until golden brown.

4. Serve with some powdered sugar, maple syrup, a dab of vegan butter and some fruit.

Maple-nut granola
Serves 20
Ingredients

½ cup raisins

½ cup dried cranberries

¼ cup canola oil

½ cup water

½ cup maple syrup

1/3 cup unsalted sunflower seeds

1/3 cup unsalted pumpkin seeds

½ cup light brown sugar

½ cup chopped pecans

½ cup sliced almonds

1 cup unsweetened coconut chips

5 cups old-fashioned rolled oats

Directions

1. Preheat the oven to 275 degrees F.

2. Combine the sunflower seeds, pumpkin seeds, brown sugar, pecans, almonds, coconut, and oats in a large bowl. Combine the oil, water, and syrup in a medium bowl.

3. Pour the wet mixture over the oat mixture and stir until well mixed.

4. Spread the mixture on a rimmed baking sheet and bake for 45 minutes.

5. Remove from the oven, stir, and continue to bake until golden brown; this should take about 45 minutes.

6. Stir in the raisins and cranberries and allow to cool before you store. Serve with your favorite non-dairy milk.

Main Courses

Avocado quinoa bowl

Servings; 2

Ingredients

1 cup of Arugula

1 cup of Brussels sprouts

½ cup quinoa

½ avocado sliced

1 tablespoon of pepitas

1 teaspoon olive oil

1 tablespoon tahini

Salt and pepper to taste

Directions

1. Cook the quinoa (follow the instructions on the packaging).

2. Sauté the Brussels sprouts for 15 minutes or until lightly browned and tender.

3. Slice the half avocado

4. Mix the arugula, cooked quinoa, Brussels sprouts, pepitas and avocado in a large bowl

5. Drizzle tahini or tahini sauce. Serve and enjoy.

Three-Bean salad

Yields 5 cups

Ingredients

For the salad

1/3 cup packed finely chopped fresh parsley

1 jalapeno, seeded and chopped (optional)

1 orange bell pepper, finely chopped

1 (15 ounce) can red kidney beans

1 (15 ounce) can chickpeas

3 finely chopped green onions

1 cup chopped green beans, stems removed

Salt and pepper to taste

For the dressing

¼ teaspoon fine grain sea salt

1 tablespoon Dijon mustard

1 tablespoon maple syrup

1 tablespoon apple cider vinegar

1 ½ tablespoon extra-virgin olive oil

8 tablespoons lemon juice

Directions

1. Add several cups of water to a pot and boil. Add the green beans and blanch them for 2 minutes in the hot water. Drain and rinse the beans with cold water then put in a large bowl.

2. Drain and rinse the kidney beans and chickpeas and place ten in the large bowl with green beans, green onion, parsley, jalapeno and bell pepper; mix.

3. Whisk the ingredients for the dressing in a small bowl until combined.

4. Pour the dressing over the salad and mix. Refrigerate for around 30 minutes to allow the flavor to develop. Season with pepper and salt and enjoy.

Spiralized Asian quinoa salad with peanut dressing

Serves 2-3

Ingredients

1/3 cup dry quinoa

1 large carrot peeled

1 teaspoon oil

2 cucumbers

¼ cup green onions, sliced (for topping)

1 cup shelled Edamame

1 tablespoon olive oil

1 ½ tablespoons soy sauce

3 tablespoons peanut butter

1 teaspoon rice wine vinegar

1 tablespoon sesame oil

1 teaspoon agave nectar

1 clove garlic (minced)

¼ teaspoon salt

Dash of ground black pepper

Directions

1. Heat some oil in a small saucepan over medium heat.

2. Add quinoa and cook for 1 minute, and then add 2/3 cup of water and bring it to boil, cover and then simmer over low heat.

3. Cook for 13-15 minutes until quinoa is cooked and fluffy.

4. Spiralize the carrots and cucumbers and place in large bowl. Add the Edamame, quinoa and green onions to the bowl and toss to combine.

5. Place the peanut butter, soy sauce, olive oil, sesame oil, vinegar, agave, garlic, salt and pepper in a blender. Blend until smooth.

6. Pour dressing over the salad and toss to combine.

Chickpea salad

Serves 3

Ingredients

1 (15 ounce) can drained chickpeas

3 green onions, sliced

2 stalks celery, chopped finely

¼ cup finely chopped red bell pepper

¼ cup finely chopped dill pickle

1 clove garlic (minced)

1 ½ teaspoons yellow mustard

3 tablespoons vegan mayonnaise

¼ teaspoon fine sea salt

Freshly ground black pepper

1 ½ -3 teaspoon fresh lemon juice

2 teaspoons minced dill (optional)

Directions

1. Mash the chickpeas in a large bowl using a potato smasher.

2. Add the green onions, pickles, bell peppers, celery, mayonnaise, garlic and stir until combined.

3. Stir in the mustard and dill, season with salt, pepper, and lemon juice to taste.

4. Serve with wraps, crackers, toasted bread or on top of a leafy green salad. You could also enjoy it on its own.

Sweet potato and beans

Serves 2

Ingredients

2 medium sized sweet potatoes

1 bunch kale

1 can black beans (drained and rinsed)

1 clove of garlic (minced)

1 tablespoon extra-virgin olive oil

Salt and pepper to taste

Dressing to serve

Directions

1. Preheat the oven to 375 degrees F.

2. Line a baking sheet with parchment paper.

3. Poke multiple holes in both sweet potatoes using a folk.

4. Bake the potatoes in an oven for 45-60 minutes.

5. Meanwhile, heat the olive oil in a skillet over medium heat. Add garlic and cook until fragrant but before it browns. Add kale and toss to coat, and then add 1/3 cup of water and cover, letting it cook for 5 minutes.

6. Uncover, toss the kales, reduce the heat, and let it cook for 15 minutes until the kale is of a desired texture. You can add water as needed.

7. Add beans to the kales and cook; season with pepper and salt and then heat until warm.

8. Cut the sweet potatoes in half lengthwise and top with the black beans and kale.

Sesame Noodles

Serves 8

Ingredients

1 pound whole-wheat spaghetti

½ cup toasted sesame seeds

1 red bell pepper, thinly sliced

4 cups snow peas, trimmed and sliced

¼ cup chopped cilantro, divided

1 bunch scallions, sliced and divided

1 ½ teaspoons crushed red pepper

2 tablespoons rice-wine vinegar

2 tablespoons canola oil

2 tablespoons sesame oil

½ cup reduced-sodium soy sauce

Directions

1. Bring a pot of water to boil, cook the spaghetti for around 9-11 minutes or until tender. Drain and rinse under running cold water.

2. Meanwhile whisk sesame oil, soy sauce, vinegar, canola oil, 2 tablespoons cilantro, ¼ cup scallions and crushed red pepper. Add the snow peas, bell pepper and noodles then toss to coat.

3. To serve, add in the sesame seeds and mix, and then garnish with the remaining cilantro and scallions.

Vegetable Soup

Serves 6-8

Ingredients

2 tablespoons chopped fresh parsley

1 teaspoon sea salt

½ teaspoon cracked black pepper

2 cups cauliflower florets, chopped

2 cups peeled butternut squash, chopped

1 large sweet potato, chopped

2 minced garlic cloves

2 chopped celery stalks

2 carrots, peeled and chopped

1 large onion, chopped

1 tablespoon olive oil

2 teaspoons Italian seasoning

6 cups vegetable stock

1 (28 ounce) can diced tomatoes

2 cups sliced cabbage

Directions

1. Heat the olive oil in a large pot over medium heat.

2. Add in the onions, celery and carrot and cook for 3 minutes or until the onions are translucent.

3. Add the garlic and cook for about a minute, and then add in cauliflower, butternut squash, and sweet potato and cook for 5 minutes.

4. Add in the tomatoes, cabbage, stock, and spices, stir and bring to a boil. Lower the heat and simmer while uncovered for around 30 minutes.

5. Top with parsley and serve warm.

Bean and rice soup
Serves 6

Ingredients

1 tablespoon sunflower oil

2 garlic cloves, minced

1 medium onion chopped

2 carrots, chopped

2 stalks celery, chopped

4 teaspoons paprika

½ cup tomato paste

2 teaspoons dried thyme

2 bay leaves

3 cups tomato juice

3 cups vegetable bouillon

1 small seeded and chopped red bell pepper

1 small seeded and chopped green bell pepper

1 (15-ounce) can of coconut milk

1 (15 ounce) can of red kidney beans

½ cup long- grain rice

3 cups day-old cubes

Sea salt and black pepper for the croutons

2 tablespoons olive oil

Directions

1. In a large saucepan, heat the oil.

2. Add the onion and cook for 5-7 minutes over medium heat until soft.

3. Add the celery, garlic, peppers, carrots, bay leaves, 2 teaspoons paprika, and cook for 5 minutes.

4. Add tomato paste, tomato juice, thyme leaves, stir, and cook for 5 minutes.

5. Stir in the bouillon, rice, and coconut milk, bring to boil, and then lower the heat to simmer for 30 minutes.

6. Add in the kidney beans and cook for 15 minutes.

7. Remove the bay leaves and season with pepper and salt, and garnish with croutons.

8. To make the croutons, toss the olive oil, 2 teaspoons paprika, stale bread and thyme, spread them in a single layer on a baking sheet and bake at 375 degrees F for 5 minutes until golden brown. Serve.

Snacks

Chickpea wraps

Serves 3-4

Ingredients

Dressing + salad

1 head romaine lettuce/1 bundle clean roughly chopped kales

1 ½ tablespoons maple syrup

1 small lemon, juiced

1-2 tablespoons hot water to thin

¼ cup + 2 tablespoons hummus

Buffalo Chickpeas

1 ¼ cups drained chickpeas

4 tablespoons hot sauce, divided

¼ teaspoon garlic powder

1 tablespoon coconut or olive oil

Pinch sea salt

For Serving

3-4 vegan friendly flour tortillas, flatbread or pita

¼ cup red onion diced

¼ cup ripe avocado, sliced

¼ cup baby tomato, diced

Directions

1. To make the dressing, mix the humus, maple syrup, and lemon juice in a mixing bowl. You can add hot water to thin the dressing.

2. Add the romaine lettuce/kale and toss. Adjust flavor as needed and set aside.

3. Add the dried chickpeas to coconut oil, 3 tablespoons hot sauce, garlic powder and pinch of salt; toss to combine.

4. Heat a skillet over medium heat; add the chickpeas and sauté for 3-5 minutes.

5. Mash a few chickpeas gently with a spoon.

6. Remove from heat once hot and slightly dried out, add remaining 1 tablespoon of hot sauce, stir to combine and set aside.

7. To assemble; top each wrap with the dressed romaine salad, ¼ cup buffalo chickpeas, sprinkle some diced tomatoes, avocado and onions. Serve

This meal can be refrigerated for up to 3 days.

Veggie Chilli

Serves 2

Ingredients

1 ready to eat mixed grain pouch

1 can chopped tomatoes

1 can kidney beans in chilli sauce

400g pack oven-roasted vegetables

Directions

1. Preheat the oven to 200 degrees Celsius. Cook the vegetables in a casserole dish for around 15 minutes.

2. Tip in the tomatoes and beans, season and cook for another 15 minutes until hot.

3. Heat the grain pouch in the oven for a minute, and then serve with the chilli.

Apple Green Smoothie

Serves 1

Ingredients

1 cup almond milk

Pinch of salt

1/8 teaspoon ground cinnamon

¼ teaspoon vanilla extract

2 medjool dates, pitted

2 cups spinach

1 frozen apple, chopped

2 ice cubes

Directions

1. Put all ingredients in your blender, blend for 30 seconds, and then serve.

Chilled Cantaloupe Soup

Serves 4

Ingredients

1 chilled cantaloupe, seeded and cut into 1-inch thick chunks

4 lime wedges

1/3 cup orange juice

Directions

1. Place the cantaloupe in a blender, add the orange juice, and blend until smooth.

2. Divide the soup among 4 bowls, squeeze lime wedges over the soup, and then serve chilled.

Mint Chocolate Smoothie

Serves 1

Ingredients

3 tablespoons non-dairy chocolate chips, divided

2 tablespoons hemp hearts

1 medium frozen banana

2 cups spinach

½ cup unsweetened rice milk

1 peppermint tea bag

½ cup boiling water

6 ice cubes

Directions

1. Steep the tea in the boiling water until it is concentrated. Let the tea cool for about 30 minutes.

2. Place all the ingredients into your blender except the chocolate chips and blend until smooth.

3. Add in half the chocolate chips and pulse quickly.

4. Pour the smoothie into a cup and top with the remaining chocolate chips.

Fruit Tart with Caramel Almond Filling

Serves 4

Ingredients

For the crust

2 cups of raisins

2 cups of walnuts

For the filling

Water, if needed

½ teaspoon of cinnamon

¼ cup of maple syrup or ½ cup of date paste

¼ cup of melted coconut oil

¼ cup of almond butter

For the topping

½ cup of goji berries

3 cups of frozen berries

Directions

1. Start by making the crust: simply pulse the walnuts in a food processor until you have a rough flour. Then add the raisins and proceed to process until it is nicely stuck together forming a fairly rough dough.

2. Press the dough into a tart tin. Next, place everything into the fridge then let it set for about 2 hours.

3. To make the filling, simply blend all the ingredients until everything is smooth.

4. Spread everything gently at the bottom of your tart crust and then allow this to harden in the fridge for about 45 minutes. Top the tart off with the berries, and slice before serving.

Desserts

Chocolate raspberry smoothie

Serves 1

Ingredients

1 cup coconut milk

1-3 ice cubes

1 tablespoon cacao powder

2 tablespoons shredded coconut

2 tablespoons ground flaxseed

1 cup raspberries

2 cups organic spinach

Directions

1. Place all the ingredients in a blender, blend until smooth, and serve.

Piña Colada Smoothie

Serves 3

Ingredients

1 (20 ounces) can crushed pineapple in juice

3 frozen bananas, peeled

1 (13.5 ounces) can coconut milk

Directions

1. Place all the ingredients in a blender and process until smooth.

2. Serve and garnish with a slice of pineapple.

Banana berry smoothie

Serves 3

Ingredients

1 ripe banana

½ cup silken tofu

1 cup frozen berries (blueberries, blackberries, raspberries)

2 ice cubes (crushed)

1 tablespoon sugar

Directions

1. Place the ice cubes in a heavy-duty plastic bag and use a roller pin to break them

2. Combine the berries, bananas, tofu, sugar and ice cubes in a blender. Blend until smooth and frothy.

Peanut Butter S'moreos

Serves 10

Ingredients

5 tablespoons of natural creamy peanut butter (ensure it is slightly warmed until pourable

10 marshmallows (vegan friendly)

20 Oreos (you can look for gluten free varieties if you want)

Directions

1. Start by placing an oven rack on the second highest position then preheat the oven to high broil.

2. Place ten Oreos onto a baking sheet then top this up with a marshmallow (or even several minis).

3. Broil on high heat for about 1-3 minutes ensuring to watch closely until it is toasted and with a deep golden brown color

4. Once deep golden brown in color, remove from the oven and then top each of the 10 using ½ tablespoon of peanut butter (ensure to warm this briefly in a

microwave if it is not pourable) and then top this with another Oreo.

Serve immediately.

Note: Popular marshmallow brands that are vegan friendly are Sweet and Sara and Dandies

Peanut Butter Fudge

Serves: 8

Ingredients

¼ teaspoon of salt

¼ teaspoon vanilla extract

2 tablespoons of maple syrup

2 tablespoons of coconut oil, melted or softened

½ cup natural peanut butter (or any natural nut butter like sunflower seed, cashew, or almond)

Directions

1. Start by combining all the ingredients in a bowl and then stir until they are well combined. To make it a little smoother,

you could microwave it in a bowl if it is hard to mix.

2. Pour the fudge into a container that has been lined with parchment paper or plastic wrap, place the container into a freezer then let it set in 30-40 minutes.

3. After it has hardened, remove from the freezer then let it sit for about 5 minutes.

4. To serve, cut with a sharp knife into 8 squares then serve immediately or store in the freezer until you are ready to eat.

30. Vegan Chocolate Milkshake

Serves: 4 small or 2 large servings
Ingredients

1 ½ cups of almond milk (you could use hemp or soy milk)

¼ cup of almond butter

2 pitted medjool dates

2 tablespoons of unsweetened cocoa powder

2 ripe medium and large bananas that are peeled, chopped into small pieces and frozen

Directions

1. Blend the ingredients until everything is smooth ensuring to add a little more almond milk whenever necessary then serve.

Conclusion

Thank you again for downloading this book!

I hope this book was able to inspire you to maintain a healthy, high protein vegan diet.

The next step is to stick to this nutritious diet and maintain a healthy lifestyle.

Part 2

Introduction

Upgrading an eating routine and way of life is no mean accomplishment.

The withdrawal manifestations backslide, and late night cooler dates are a horrible truth of eating less.

Indeed, even the most propelled, eager individuals can fall at the significant jump with regards to changing over to a Vegan eat less.

The charming allurement of nourishments like bacon or cheddar (for instance) is in some cases excessively.

Things being what they are, how might you begin another sound way of life without the need to go after that burger?

That is the thing that I am will discuss today.

This book loaded with supportive tips and techniques for natural; home cooked meals which are vegan, healthy and easy to prepare.

The recipes in Isa Does It are supermarket friendly and don't have any exotic ingredients.

It is a great vegan cookbook for beginners who are on a tight schedule.

The recipes intended for those with occupied timetables, working mothers, and determined workers, with the expectation to make a veggie lover way of life as open as could be expected under the circumstances.

A portion of the formulas highlighted in this book are:

- Red Hot Red Pepper Salsa
- Loco Lo Mien
- Joe Allen's Polka Pepper Pasta
- Lime Splashed Butternut Squash over Rice
- Peanut Topped Greens
- Rich roasted eggplant
- Potato skin fry

None of these formulas are confounded or tedious - they made for individuals who are working all day, or even only the individuals who aren't incredibly sure about the kitchen.

This cookbook is brimming with formulas which will speak to veggie lovers as well as health-conscious people too.

Chalupas

Commands to make your precise personal chalupas with shells that are clean outwardly and uncooked within. These shells maintain as much as a considerable degree of filling.

Ingredients

18 little corn tortillas (around three creeps in distance throughout) or larger corn tortillas attacked comparable shapes

Half container sunflower oil for broiling one glass refried beans

Two (2) carrots, bubbled or steamed and hacked

Two (2) little beets, bubbled or steamed and slashed half of the onion, daintily reduce

Six (6) radishes, slashed

Three (3) tbsp cilantro (coriander) or parsley slashed one field destroyed lettuce

Salsa from a jug or maybe better, and handcrafted Sea salt to taste.

Instructions

Sear the two aspects of the tortilla within the warmed oil till firm. Deplete on paper towels and orchestrate on a plate. Unfold tortilla with refried beans and cowl with carrots, beets, onion, radishes, cilantro, lettuce, salsa and salt to flavor.

Ron's Best Guacamole

Guacamole can be set up in two courses: with a bowl and fork or in the molcajete, a Mexican mortar, and pestle. Making it in the molcajete gets the most amazing outcomes. This method is the best

Ingredients

Three (3) very ripe avocados smashed with a fork

Four (4) fresh jalapeno chiles, seeded and finely slashed juice of 2 limes.

1/2 tsp salt

Instructions

Blend the avocado with the chiles, include the lime juice and salt, mix well and serve with tortilla chips.

Jicama con Limon y Chile

A refreshing, healthy and delicious snack. My children love it, so I like to prepare it at home to avoid eaten on the street.

Ingredients

One lb jicama, peeled and cut into 1/4 inch slices juice of 5 green limes or 2 lemons

1/2 tsp powdered chile pequin (or Spanish smoked pimenton) fine grain sea salt to taste

Instructions

Set up the jicama slices on a platter. Sprinkle the lime juice at the top, observed with the aid of the chile and salt. Simple and non-fat!

Sopa de Nopal (Cactus Soup)

Cactus stew from Mexico its proper preparation for dinner Susana Rangel Gutierrez flavored with crispy pork rinds, which add robust depth and crunch.

Ingredients

8oz can nopalitos

1 quart boiling salted water 1/8 tsp baking soda

Two whole cloves garlic one small onion, sliced

2 lb green tomatillos, roasted in a skillet 1-quart water

One chipotle chile 1/2 tsp marjoram

Instructions

Roast the tomatos in a skillet for 5 minutes, turning occasionally. Blend the tomatillos with the garlic an 1 cup of the water. Strain and add the nopalitos, the chipotle chile, adding three more cups of water.

Add the marjor ingredints, and bring to a boil, after that put salt to the taste. Now you can serve with tortillas warmed in a dry skillet, wrapped in a cloth napkin.

Tequila Avocado Soup

Avocado soup with a splash of tequila— an excellent way to mention 'Viva Mexico!' Why try? Did soup make with tequila? C'mon, that's something worth trying. Serve with a salad for a light and relaxed summer season supper.

Ingredients

Four medium avocados, cut in half, pits removed, and pulp scooped out

Two tablespoons tequila

3 1/2 cups chicken broth

2/3 cup half and half

One tablespoon finely chopped green onion or scallion

1/2 tablespoon hot sauce

Salt to taste

Instructions

1 is all elements, besides salt, in a blender or food processor and liquefy till smooth, doing this in two batches if necessary.

Two taste for seasoning, upload salt and pulse in brief.

Three Refrigerate one hour before serving.

4 Garnish with chopped tomatoes, corn and crumbled Viscount St. Albans. Served chilled.

Textured Vegetable Protein Mole Enchiladas

If I had a single preferred food, mole might be it. It's the right mixture of candy and savory, and its super intensity of flavor will confuse the crap out of your palette while delighting it.

Ingredients

2 cups Red Mole Sauce (see below)

1/3 cup olive oil

Six cloves garlic, peeled 1/2 onion finely chopped

One 1/2 cups textured vegetable protein granules soaked for 10 minutes in 1 1/4 cups water or vegetable stock

1/2 tsp thyme 1/2 tsp cumin one tsp salt

12 corn tortillas

Instructions

Prepare the Mole Sauce. Even as it's cooking, warm the olive oil and sauté the garlic and onion for 5 minutes. Add the soaked textured vegetable protein, thyme, cumin and salt, and stir well to combine over low heat.

Heat the tortillas one after the other on a hot comal or dry skillet, then dip in the Red Mole Sauce until soft. Place on a working plate, place a small amount of the seasoned textured vegetable protein in the middle and roll into a tube. Arrange the filled tortillas in an ovenproof dish until ready to serve anytime. Warm for 10-15 minutes in a 375F oven befor serving. Place two on each plate and cover with more sauce. Serve with Mexican rice and a salad.

Red Mole Sauce (makes 2 cups)

Red mole is a Mexican sauce that comes in about as many varieties as there are households in the country. Puebla and Oaxaca are two regions known for their moles with varieties including Verde (green), Negro (black), and Rojo (red).

Ingredients

Four ancho chilies, roasted and seeded

Two tomatoes, roasted, peeled and seeded five cloves of garlic, roasted and peeled 1/3 cup almonds

1/3 cup peanuts 1/3 cup raisins

One slice of toasted bread three green onions chopped one tsp sea salt water

1/4 cup sesame or corn oil

Instructions

The traditional Mexican way to roast the chile, tomatoes and garlic are on a hot comal. You may also bake them in a dry skillet, turning to scorch on all sides. Some American chefs roast them beneath the appliance within the oven. After roasting combination all the components besides the oil with sufficient water to make a thick sauce. Heat the oil in a heavy saucepan and upload the sauce. Cook 20 minutes add water to thin the sauce as preferred.

Mexican Rice with Vegetables

Mexican Rice with Vegetables: serve is as a side or as the main dish with tacos, burritos & more. Vegan & gluten free.

Ingredients

1/2 cup sunflower oil

One clove garlic

3 cups (2 lbs) rice

One onion, sliced

Two small tomatoes, peeled, seeded and chopped one poblano chile, cut into strips

One medium zucchini, cut into pieces

Two carrots cut into strips

One chayote, cut into strips or 1/2 cup peas 4 cups hot water

Salt to taste one tsp pepper

One sprig fresh thyme

Instructions

Warm the oil in 1 1/2 quart pot with a tight-fitting lid. Brown the garlic and rice for about 10-15 minutes. Add the onion and tomatoes and brown with the rice for five more minutes. Add the chile, zucchini and chayote (or peas) and brown for two more minutes. Add the water, salt, black pepper, and thyme, and bring to a boil. Lower the heat, cover with a tight-fitting lid and simmer for another 20 minutes.

Stuffed cabbage in chipotle sauce

Have you ever had crammed cabbage rolls with sauerkraut? It's a traditional Hungarian dish. Gently cooked large cabbage leaves stuffed with a mixture of paprika-spiced ground pork, onions, and garlic, and then rolled up into little bundles.

Ingredients

One head of cabbage

1 cups of cooked rice 1 tbsp garlic, chopped

1/4 cup almonds, blanched and peeled 1/4 cup sliced green olives

1/4 cup parsley, chopped one tsp thyme

1/4 cup chopped zucchini sea salt to taste

Chipotle sauce:

Four medium tomatoes, roasted

Three chipotle chiles seeded and washed two cloves of garlic

Salt to taste

Instructions

Remove the center core and outer leaves from 1 head of cabbage and drop it into boiling water. Carry out after a couple of minutes and dispose of the soft sheets. Repeat, in the process cut the head and removing leaves until you have successfully separated 12 of them.

In a large bowl, mix the rice, garlic, almonds, olives, parsley, thyme, zucchini, and salt. Put a portion of this mixture into the middle of each cabbage leaf, fold the sides over and then roll them up into a packet. Preheat the oven to 375F.

To prepare the sauce, put the tomatoes, chilies, and garlic in a blender and puree and strain. Add the salt to taste. Place the sauce over the cabbage rolls, and cover to bake for 20 minutes.

Chiles Rellenos

Chiles Rellenos", a dish that requires a while and skill within the kitchen due to its complexity. Doña Rosa tells that someday her husband got here back early from work and noticed her on the manner to the market.

Ingredients

12 poblano chiles Picadillo filling:

One head of garlic 1 tbsp oregano 1/8 tsp cloves 1/4 tsp cinnamon

1/4 tsp black pepper half tsp sea salt

Two (2) tbsp sparkling squeezed orange juice 2 tbsp apple cider vinegar

Two (2) cups textured vegetable protein granules 4 tbsp olive oil

One red onion chopped four tomatoes

15 green olives, chopped 20 raisins

1/2 cup croutons

1 cup salsa

Instructions

Roast the chilies on a comal or in a large, dry skillet. While they are still hot, place them in a plastic bag to sweat until cooled. Place them in a full pan with clean water and rub it off the scorched skin. chile to remove the veins and the seeds. Rinse well. Roast and peel the garlic.

To make the filling, blend the garlic, oregano, cloves cinnamon, black pepper, salt, orange juice, and vinegar. Hydrate the textured vegetable protein granules in 1 3/4 cup hot water, stirring to moisten evenly. Roast, peel, seed and chop the tomatoes. Heat the oil and sauté the onion for 5 minutes. Add the tomatoes and continue to sauté for ten more minutes. Adding the green olives and the raisins, stir and combine with the textured vegetable protein. Turn off heat. Preheat the oven to 350F. Stuff the chiles with the picadillo filling. Arrange in an ovenproof dish and top with croutons. Bake for 20 minutes and serve with warmed salsa.

Chiles Rellenos Stuffed with Brown Rice

I love chiles. I mean really, they make everything taste better whether it be pasta dishes, scrambled eggs, and even pizza. I love 'em! And I love chile rellenos but the batter on them is fattening and usually thick and soggy, which is a total drag, so I like to make stuffed poblano chiles with different things in them like ground beef or turkey, but these are vegetarian.

Ingredients

Four large poblano chilies or 3 small ones, peeled, seeded and deveined (see below)
3 cups cooked brown rice

1/4 cup fresh cilantro/coriander or parsley, chopped four green onions, chopped

1/2 tsp salt

2 cups refried beans 1 cup water

1-pint vegan sour 'cream' (Tofutti brand or make your own) 1/2 cup green onions, chopped

Instructions

Preheat the oven to 375F. To peel the chilies, first, roast them on a hot grill or under the broiler, occasionally turning until they blistered. Place all in a plastic bag to sweat for little time, then peel. And Cut a slit down the side of each chile. Remove the seeds and the veins with care (you may want to wear gloves).

Combine the rice, cilantro/coriander, green onions and salt and fill the chiles with this mixture. Arrange the chiles in a lightly oiled 9x9inch baking dish and bake for 20 minutes. Make a sauce by heating the refried beans with the water, mixing well over low heat while the chilies cook.

To serve, spoon the bean sauce over each chile and garnish with a spoonful of sour 'cream' and some chopped green onions.

Salsa Mexicana

The complimentary chips and salsa were fresh and delicious, with an assortment of hot, mild and salsa verde. I wanted a salad that wasn't on the menu, and they were very accommodating, and it was yummy. I had a margarita that was so good.

Ingredients

3 tbsp fresh jalapeno chilies, and chopped

Three Italian (Roma) of tomatoes or 2 large round ones, chopped 1 tbsp fresh cilantro/coriander, chopped

juice of 1 lime

1/4 tsp finely ground sea salt Combine ingredients and serve. Salsa Tapatio

Eight dried de Arbol chiles (or any small dried chilies) 3 fat cloves garlic, peeled

juice of 2 limes

1/2 tsp finely ground salt or to taste spring water to thin

Instructions

Roast the chilies in a dry skillet over medium heat for 5 minutes with the window open (otherwise, the vapors may irritate nose and eyes). Grind them with the garlic in a molcajete if you have one or better use a blender. Add the lime juice, and some water to keep it fluid, keep grinding or blending, add the salt and strain. Prepare ahead before time. It keeps well in sterilized jars in the refrigerator.

Banana Flambé

Bananas flambé makes an impressive presentation with the lights off because rum is flamed to finish this simple banana dessert dish favorite in the French Caribbean.

Ingredients

2 tbsp brown sugar one tsp cinnamon

2 tbsp margarine

Six ripe bananas, peeled and sliced in half, lengthwise 3 tbsp dark Caribbean rum

Instructions

Mix the brown sugar and cinnamon. Preheat the oven to 400F. Grease a 9x12inch ovenproof dish with margarine and sprinkle with half the cinnamon/brown sugar mixture. Arrange the bananas in the bowl with the cutting style side down the Sprinkle with the rest of the cinnamon sugar mix and dot with margarine. Bake about 10 minutes or until the bananas are well cooked. Remove from the oven, sprinkle with the rum and ignite. Serve hot with vegan ice 'cream.'

Salsa Chipotle

Acquire knowledge to make authentic Chipotle Hot Salsa with roasted tomatillos and spicy red chiles. It only takes five ingredients to get up this copycat recipe at home!

Ingredients

Makes 3/4 cup

Four dried chipotle chiles 1/2 cup hot water

Two cloves garlic 1/2 tsp salt

1/4 cup apple cider vinegar

Instructions

Soke the chiles in the water for 5 minutes soften, then remove the stem and seeds. Grind them in a blender with the soaking water, garlic, salt, and vinegar. Put into a small saucepan and simmer over medium heat for 5 minutes. Let cool and pour into a jar.

Fennel a la Grecque

A simple recipe that brings out the lovely licorice flavor of the fennel. Unfortunately, the fronds were cut off the only bulb I could find so I couldn't sprinkle on top but that didn't detract from the flavor. I used ground coriander. It is a do again recipe

Ingredients

2 cups olive oil

2 cups white wine vinegar

¾ cup white wine 12 cloves garlic

One medium onion

One lemon

24 peppercorns

Four bay leaves

2 tbsp fennel seed four small bulbs fennel Method

In a big pot, bring the olive oil, vinegar and white wine to a gentle simmer.

Instructions

Peel the garlic. Peel and slice the onion very thin. Slice the lemon crosswise into ¼ inch slices and add to the pot along with the onion, garlic, peppercorns, bay leaves and fennel seed. Simmer for about 15 minutes.

Cut off the feathery tops and stalks from the fennel bulbs and remove any tight outer layers. Cut the bulbs into eighths. Add all to the simmering liquid and cook until they are tender but still slightly crunchy. Remove from pot and let them cool. When both the fennel and the liquid have cooled down finaly, return the fennel to the liquid and keep it in the refrigerator. It will be nice if it sits for 24 hours.

Caramelised Fennel

The only key that the fennel, no crowding. Cook in batches if necessary- the only problem will be that you will finish the first batch before the next batch done. Yes, this dish is that good.

Ingredients

Two large fennel bulbs

¼ cup olive oil salt and pepper

Trim the fennel bulbs, removing any tough outer layers. Cut into bulbs in half vertically, cut out the cores and cut the bulbs into 1/8 inch thick slices.

Instructions

Heat a big sauté pan over medium heat, add olive oil, and when the oil is hot, add the sliced fennel (if necessary, cook the fennel in two batches; the fennel should brown, not steam). Cook, tossing or occasionally stirring for 8-10 minutes until fennel is caramelized and tender. Season with salt and pepper. Drain off any excess oil and serve. Excellent as a side vegetable or a pizza topping.

Grilled Asparagus with Blood Oranges and Tapenade Toast

This fast, and easy recipe is an example of "spring" to me. There is no tale at the back of it, only a conventional aggregate of the fresh spring asparagus, and sweet blood oranges. So that the flavors will compliment each other, and the colors are lovely collectively at the plate.

Ingredients

One shallot

Three blood of oranges 1 ½ tsp balsamic vinegar

½ tsp red wine vinegar extra virgin olive oil salt and pepper

1 ½ pounds fat asparagus (25 –30 spears) 4 slices country-style bread

Tapenade (olives, garlic, olive oil whizzed together)

Instructions

Peel and chop the shallot finely and macerate for 30 minutes in the juice of ½ orange and the balsamic and red wine vinegar. Whisk in the olive oil up to taste to make a vinaigrette, add season with salt, and pepper all together., and Peel just the zest from one of the oranges chop it very high-quality and upload it to the French dressing.

Cut away all of the rind and pith from all the oranges and slice them crosswise into thin rounds.

Snap off the robust backside at the ends of the asparagus spears; you must Peel the spears and the parboil them in salted water for about 1 minute, till they're just soft. Spread them out to empty thoroughly and cool to room temperature. Brush with olive oil, salt lightly and grill for approximately 6 minutes over medium warmness, often turning to brown evenly. Toast bread at the equal time.

Moroccan Chickpeas

Hot Moroccan Chickpeas formula will never frustrate. A portion of the online analysts says, Great Made this for a supper party and presented with hummus and pita."

Ingredients

One glasses dried chickpeas one little carrot.

One yellow onion

One little bundle cilantro

The 2-inch handle of crisp ginger

1-inch bit of the cinnamon stick one squeeze ground saffron

½ tsp cayenne two ready tomatoes salt

Instructions

Absorb chickpeas overnight bloodless water. Peel all the carrot, and onion and slash generally. Deplete the chickpeas and cowl with clean water. Convey to a bubble, skim off the foam and swing down to a stew. Include the carrot and onion. Decrease off the stems of the cilantro and save the leaves to decorate the finished dish. Tie the stems in a package and transfer to the chickpeas close by the ginger, peeled, and the cinnamon, saffron, turmeric a cayenne. Hold the chickpeas submerged in water as they cook, however, do never again include additional water than essential, all together now not to weaken the flavourful stock.

Peel, seed coarse slash tomatoes. After 30 to forty-five mins, while the chickpeas are around 75% cooked add the tomatoes and salt to enhance. Keep on simmering until the point that the chickpeas are exceptionally delicate and the soup has thickened scarcely around 60 minutes. Take away and dispose of the cinnamon, ginger, and cilantro stems. Taste for flavoring, decorate with the saved cilantro leaves and serve over cooked couscous. Present with a dab of harissa glue.

Eggplant, Tomato and Onion Gratin

Asian eggplants are thin and prolonged. The Japanese assortment is dark purple while a Chinese variety, Asian Bride, is pale lavender. Simmering, preparing or barbecuing eggplant before adding it to a sauté shields it from getting too slick.

Ingredients

Three substantial sweet white onions three cloves garlic

Olive oil

2 or 3 sprigs thyme

One inlet leaf

Salt and pepper

Three medium Japanese eggplants three ready tomatoes

Instructions

Peel and hack the onions and garlic fine. Stew them over a medium fire for around 5 minutes until the point when delicate in several tbsp olive oil, with the leaves of the thyme, the narrows leaf and salt and pepper.

Cut the eggplant into ¼ inch rounds. Cut the tomatoes somewhat thicker. Preheat stove to 400F. Oil a shallow gratin dish.

Expel the straight leaf from the onions and spread them over the base of the dish. Cover with covering lines of interchange tomato and eggplant cuts. Each cut should cover 66% of the first one. Season with salt and pepper, sprinkle with some more olive oil, cover and cook on the stove until the point that the eggplant is sufficiently delicate to be cut with a spoon, around 45 minutes. Reveal throughout the previous 15 minutes or prior if the tomatoes are surrendering excessively fluid. Brush or spoon the juices over the best sporadically to keep the best layer from drying out. This gratin ought to be sodden however not watery.

Bean Ragout with Potato Gnocchi

Asian eggplants are slim and extended. The Japanese assortment is dull purple while a Chinese variety, Asian Bride, is pale lavender. Cooking, heating or barbecuing eggplant before adding it to a sauté shields it from getting too sleek.

Ingredients

Three substantial sweet white onions three cloves garlic

Olive oil

2 or 3 sprigs thyme

One straight leaf

Salt and pepper

Three medium Japanese eggplants three ready tomatoes

Instructions

Peel and leave the onions and garlic okay. Stew them over a medium fire for around 5 minutes until the point when delicate in two or three tbsp olive oil, with the leaves of the thyme, the sound leaf and salt and pepper.

Cut the eggplant into ¼ inch rounds. Cut the tomatoes somewhat thicker. Preheat grill to 400F. Oil a shallow gratin dish.

Expel the straight leaf from the onions and spread them over the base of the dish.

Cover with covering columns of interchange tomato and eggplant cuts. Each cut should cover 66% of the first one. Season with salt and pepper, sprinkle with some more olive oil, cover and cook on the stove until the point that the eggplant is sufficiently delicate to be cut with a spoon, around 45 minutes. Reveal throughout the previous 15 minutes or prior if the tomatoes are surrendering excessively fluid. Brush or spoon the juices over the best periodically to keep the best layer from drying out. This gratin ought to be wet yet not watery.

Potato, Morel and Onion Fricassee

This natural chicken stew highlights dried mushrooms, new potatoes, leeks, bacon and fresh herbs for a flavorful, fulfilling one-dish supper.

Ingredients

1 ½ pounds Yellow Finn or reddish brown potatoes salt and pepper

One small onion

½ pound morels 2 tbsp margarine

¼ - ½ container vegetable oil

¼ hacked parsley strategy

Instructions

All the potatoes must be peel and cut them into large pieces and bubble in salted water until the point that they are delicate and the edges have begun to separate. Be mindful so as not to overcook them, or they go into disrepair entirely. Deplete and put aside to dry. Cut the onion thin.

Cut the morels down the middle longwise and wash rapidly in a lot of water. Deplete and sauté in the margarine over a high fire. They will discharge some water. Turn the fire down to medium, let the mushrooms reabsorb their juices and keep cooking until the point that they scorched.

Broil the potatoes in a large skillet in 1/8 inch of the oil over medium warmth. At the point when the vegetables have begun to turn brilliant darker, include the cut onions. At the end when the potatoes are firm, and the onions start caramelizing channel off an abundance of oil, include the morels and the cleaved parsley, season with salt and pepper. Hurl together and serve.

Sichuan Kung Pao 'Chicken'

Zesty fowl with peanuts, like what served in Chinese eateries. It's miles whatever but hard to make, and you can be as messy with the estimations as you need. They decrease to a decent, thick sauce. Replacement cashews for peanuts, or bamboo shoots for the water chestnuts. You can not flip out severely! Respect!

Ingredients

12-14 ounces firm tofu, cut into strips 1 tbsp mild soy sauce

1 tbsp cornstarch 1/eight tsp white pepper 1 tbsp oil

four green onions, cut slantingly into 3/4 inch pieces two tsp minced garlic

1 tbsp bean stew garlic glue

One crimson ringer pepper, seeded and cut into 3/4 inch squares 1 tbsp dark colored bean glue

half glass cool veggie lover soup 1 tbsp cornstarch

One tsp light unbleached sugar

1 cup unsalted cooked peanuts or cashews, cleaved

Instructions

Combination the tofu with the soy sauce, two tsp cornstarch and white pepper. Warm a wok or massive skillet over high warmth. Each time hot, including the oil. At the point, while the oil is heated, encompass the tofu and panfry till delicately seared. Include the raw onions, garlic, and bean stew garlic glue. Panfry for 1 minute.

Consist of the chile pepper and darkish colored bean glue. Panfry for two mins.

Mix the soup, 1 tbsp cornstarch, and sugar, and upload to the dish. Combination until thickened. Sprinkle the peanuts to finish the whole lot and serve quickly with rice.

Stir-Fried Tofu with Leeks

I honestly love leek. This week we were given a bunch of fresh, natural greens from a neighborhood farmer, together with about a dozen leeks. I decided to prepare dinner a dish that centers around leek.

Ingredients

Cooking Sauce:

One tsp chili garlic paste

One half tablespoons darkish soy sauce 1 tbsp dry sherry

1/2 cup to one cup mild vegetarian broth

1 tbsp oil

Instructions

12 oz. leeks, adequately cleaned, hard leaves discarded and shredded with a pointy knife (both white and inexperienced elements) three cloves garlic, minced 12-14 oz firm tofu, sliced

into small triangles and pan-fried in 2 tbsp hot oil till golden on both aspects combine the cooking sauce ingredients in a bowl and set apart.

Warm a massive wok or heavy skillet over high heat. When it's hot, add the oil. While the oil is hot, upload the leeks and garlic. Stir-fry for approximately three minutes.

Add the tofu and the cooking sauce and cook three extra mins. Serve straight away with rice.

Vegetarian Stir Fry 'Oyster' Sauce

It is an authentic and comfortable Chinese language recipe for doing a wholesome vegetable dish without dropping any vitamins. It is easy and rapid to make and loved by using young and old alike. Oyster sauce is simple to locate in any Asian food store and most grocery stores.

Ingredients

One mushroom broth dice

1/2 cup boiling water

2 tbsp brown bean sauce

One generous tablespoon dark unbleached sugar one tsp cornstarch dissolved in 1 tsp bloodless water

Instructions

Dissolve the broth dice in the boiling water. Blend with the brown bean sauce and sugar, and warmth to boiling. Upload the dissolved cornstarch and stir until thickened. Cool and shop in a blanketed jar within the refrigerator.

Sichuan 'Beef' and Broccoli

This shellfish hamburger with broccoli can be present with steamed rice or noodles. What's more, if you want to panfry with shellfish sauce, I high prescribe utilizing Lee Kum Kee premium clam sauce.

Ingredients

1 cups reconstituted finished soy protein pieces blended with 2 tbsp dim soy sauce one tsp cornstarch

1 tbsp cooking oil

Six cloves garlic minced

One bunch of broccoli (stalks peeled) cut into thin cuts (around six containers) 1 to 2 expansive onions, each cut into six wedges, layers isolated

2 tbsp water

One large red chile pepper, seeded and cut into 1-inch squares Cooking Sauce:

1 tbsp vinegar (rice, juice or white wine) 1 tbsp bean stew garlic glue

1/2 tbsp light unbleached sugar one glass light of veggie lover stock

1 tbsp cornstarch blended with 2 tbsp ice water

Instructions

Blend the soy protein with the one tsp cornstarch. Warm the oil in a non-stick wok or large skillet over high warmth. Include the garlic and soy protein pieces. Panfry until the point when the soy protein pieces are seared. Expel from the dish and put aside.

Consolidate the cooking sauce fixings in a bowl and put aside.

Include the broccoli, onions, chile peppers and 2 tbsp water to the container. is done point that the broccoli is merely fresh delicate. Include somewhat more water if important

Include the soy protein lumps back to the skillet, alongside the cooking sauce. Mix until the point when the sauce is thickened and serve instantly.

Red Pepper Tofu

This attractive stir-fry stimulated with the aid of a traditional Chinese language dish known as rainbow pork. The vegetarian model works nicely, and it's additionally less complicated to make. In case you opt for completely firm tofu, take the more time to weight it as directed in step 1. I am satisfied to bypass this step and use company tofu that hasn't weighted.

Ingredients

12-14 oz firm or greater firm tofu reduce into half of the inch cubes three tbsp vegetarian stir fry 'oyster' sauce

1/3 cup vegetarian broth 6 tbsp dry sherry

6 tbsp light soy sauce

2 tbsp vinegar (rice, cider or white wine) three tbsp mild unbleached sugar

Four tsp chili garlic paste

1 tbsp oil vegetables:

2 tbsp minced garlic

Four stalks celery, diagonally sliced 1/four inch thick one massive crimson bell pepper, seeded and thinly sliced one medium onion, thinly sliced

four tsp cornstarch dissolved in 2 tbsp water

1/3 cup chopped toasted walnuts, almonds or cashews

Instructions

Mix the tofu cubes very well with the vegetarian stir fry 'oyster' sauce in a bowl and allow stand even as you put together the different components.

Mix the cooking sauce ingredients in a glass and set apart.

Warmness a massive wok or heavy skillet over high warmness. When hot, upload the oil. While the oil is warm, upload all of the vegetables. Stir-fry over excessive warmth for 1 minute. Add the tofu an stir-fry 1 minute more. Stir in the cooking sauce. Convey to a boil, then simmer for three mins over medium heat till the sauce thickens.

Pour onto a heated platter or shallow serving bowl and pinnacle with toasted nuts. Serve immediately.

Mapo Doufu

I cherish cooking map tofu for a quick lunch or supper. Some of the time I twofold the meat and sauce, so it will likely be sufficient to serve people as a one-dish supper. I likewise get a kick out of danger to include a modest bunch of veggies (mustard veggies or spinach) in the direction of the end of braising, to make a more nutritious and adjusted feast. I frequently supplant the ground pork (applied as a part of the credible adaptation) with ground turkey to cut calories.

Ingredients

1/2 bins water

1/4 container mild soy sauce

Four tsp stew garlic glue or 2 disintegrated dried hot bean stew peppers

1 cup dried completed soy protein granules absorbed five mins 7/eight glass bubbling water two tsp dry sherry

Two tsp soy sauce

Two tsp hoisin sauce 1/2 tbsp oil

Two tsp minced garlic

Four tsp minced crisp ginger

1 lb medium-company fresh tofu, reduce into half-inch three-D shapes and set in a colander to burn up. four green onions, meagerly reduce

4 tbsp cornstarch mixed with four tbsp frosty water

Instructions

Be part of the cooking sauce fixings in a bowl and placed apart.

Combo the doused complete soy protein with sherry, two tsp soy sauce, and hoisin sauce. Placed aside.

Warm temperature an expansive wok or overwhelming skillet over high warmth. On the point, while it's hot, consist of the oil. At the end when the oil is warm, encompass the garlic and ginger and panfry quick. Include the completed soy protein combination and panfry for two mins. Include the tofu and cooking sauce and stew for three mins.

Consist of the soft onions and the cornstarch mixture and mix over excessive warmth until thick and bubbly. Serve promptly.

Hunan Hot and Sour Vegetarian "Duck"

This warm and cruel soup is the maximum credible take-out warm and sharp soup you've got ever had and route superior to

Chinese language take-out spots. See together with your own eyes!

Ingredients

Two 10oz jars veggie lover "broil duck" gluten (seitan) (mun chaitya) 1 tbsp oil

One little green pepper, seeded and reduce into 1-inch squares 1/2 box reduce celery

1/2 box meagerly cut carrots

1 tbsp aged darkish beans, squashed with a fork half tbsp minced garlic

1 tbsp new floor ginger one tsp bean stew garlic glue

1 cup veggie lover stock 2 tbsp light soy sauce

2 tbsp rice, juice or white wine vinegar 2 tbsp dry sherry

One tsp cornstarch broke down in 1 tbsp cold water

Instructions

Wash the gluten in a colander and cut it into chomp measure pieces. Warmth an expansive wok or overwhelming skillet over excessive warm temperature until extraordinarily warm. Encompass the oil. On the factor when the oil is heated, consist of the gluten and panfry for a few minutes.

Consist of the vegetables, darkish beans, garlic, ginger, stew garlic glue, and soup. Bubble for 1 minute. Include soy sauce, vinegar and sherry, turn down the warmth and stew for four to six minutes. Consist of the disintegrated cornstarch and mix until thickened. Serve right away.

Steamed Tofu with Spicy Bean Paste Sauce

I've heard the protest on limitless occasions: tofu is excessively flat. In place of considering it to be an imperfection, be that as it may, I keep minding it to be first-rate. The lack of bias of tofu makes it the perfect sustenance to ingest different flavors, individually solid ones, as salted dark beans, which mortgage an unmistakably impactful, smoky taste to this system. Serve this dish with steamed darkish colored rice for an honestly delicious and sound dinner.

Ingredients

Sixteen oz.medium-firm tofu

1 tbsp oil

One liberal tbsp cleaved inexperienced onions 1/2 tbsp minced crisp ginger

1/2 tbsp minced garlic

One half of tbsp Sichuan hot bean glue or dark colored bean glue with stew garlic glue added to the flavor

2 tbsp in addition to two tsp mild soy sauce 2/three box vegan soup

One liberal tsp cornstarch broke up in 1 tbsp icy water 1/2 tbsp broiled sesame oil

Discretionary: 1 tbsp new cilantro

Slice the tofu into four squares. Steam the squares over carbonated water for 10 minutes.

Instructions

While the tofu steams, installation the sauce. It is going brief so have the whole thing hacked and anticipated. warmth a wok or giant skillet over high warm temperature. On the point, while it is hot, encompass the oil. On end, while the oil is hot, consist of the soft onion, ginger, garlic and bean glue. Blend for 10 seconds. Encompass the soy sauce and soup and warmth to the point of boiling. The mixture inside the broke up cornstarch and encompass the sesame oil. Take the dish off the heat.

Deplete the tofu in a colander. Cut the empty squares into 1-inch squares and orchestrate them correctly on a warmed serving bowl. Pour the sauce over the squares and sprinkle it with cilantro.

Hunan Style "Duck" Curry

Clean smell and deep tones. Usual cooking strategies incorporate stewing, broiling, pot-simmering, braising and smoking. Given the high farming yield of the place, elements for Hunan dishes are numerous and differed.

Ingredients

1 tbsp oil

1 to 2 jars veggie lover "Broil Duck" braised gluten seitan (mun chaitya) or ridicule duck, washed and cut into 1-inch parcels

3 tbsp curry glue or powder 2 tbsp minced garlic

Two tsp ground new ginger half tsp stew garlic glue

One substantial unpracticed pepper, cut into 1-inch squares

1/4 to half of the lb of mushrooms, split (utilize best 50% of pound on the off chance that you just use one jar of "duck") 1 expansive onion, peeled, cut into six wedges, layers isolated

2 cups veggie lover juices 1/four container mellow soy sauce 1/4 glass dry sherry

2 tbsp cornstarch broke up in 2 tbsp frosty water

Instructions

Warm a considerable work or substantial skillet over extreme warmth. While it's boiling, include the oil. While the oil is hot, include the seitan, curry, garlic, ginger and stew glue. Panfry for 1-2 minutes, at that point, add the green pepper and Mushrooms and onion. Panfry for some other 2 minutes.

Include the stock, soy sauce, and sherry. Cowl, flip the glow the distance down to medium-low and stew for 10 minutes. Blend inside the disintegrated cornstarch, turn the warmth as much as high and mix until the point when it has thickened.

Present with steamed rice.

Hunan Tofu with Fresh Garlic

A quite hot (or extraordinarily fiery on the off danger which you like) eggplant dish. My mom has been making this for me because I used to be a tyke. It is appropriate!!

Ingredients

6 to 7 additional company tofu

One tsp mild soy sauce one tsp dry sherry

One tsp cornstarch

1 tbsp oil

2 tbsp minced crisp garlic

1/2 massive green pepper, seeded and reduce into squares 1/2 glass diced celery

Two carrots, cleaned and meagerly reduce on the corner to corner half glass veggie lover juices

1 tbsp dry sherry

2 tbsp light soy sauce

Two tsp cornstarch broke down in 2 tbsp frosty water

Reduce the tofu into three/four inch squares, 1/4 inch thick. Mixture the squares in a bowl with the one tsp soy sauce, one tsp sherry, and one tsp cornstarch.

Instructions

Warmth a sizeable wok or sizeable skillet over excessive heat until notably hot.

Include the oil. At the point, while the oil is hot, include the tofu. Panfry until the point that it begins to darker. Encompass the garlic, pepper, celery, and carrots and panfry for three to five minutes. Include the stock and cook for 1 minute. Encompass the 1 tbsp sherry, 2 tbsp soy sauce and the broke up cornstarch and mix until the factor that it thickens. Serve promptly.

Chinese-Style Chili Green Beans

Spicy Chinese language Sichuan green Beans are an appropriate smooth side dish on your favorite Chinese language meal, and they're a breeze to make with just a few components.

Ingredients

1 lb small fresh green beans, trimmed or frozen small whole inexperienced beans (Do no longer use frozen reduce berries for this dish!)

1 tbsp oil

Two cloves garlic, crushed

Half tsp dried crimson chili flakes 2 tbsp mild soy sauce

1/2 tsp unrefined sugar one tsp roasted sesame oil

Instructions

In case you are the usage of fresh beans, blanch them for approximately 2 minutes in boiling water, then drain and vicinity them in cold water. If the usage of frozen berries, thaw them in a colander by using running hot water over them. Drain the beans well.

Warm a big wok or heavy skillet over excessive warmness. When it's warm, upload the oil and flip the heat all the way down to medium. Upload the garlic and chili flakes and stir-fry for a minute. Add the green beans, soy sauce, and sugar and flip up the heat to excessive. Stir-fry for 3-5 mins until the seeds finished. Sprinkle with the sesame oil and serve. Those beans are also incredible while served at room temperature.

Chinese-Style Zucchini with Ginger

Darkish bean sauce, ginger, and Thai chilies make this zucchini an excellent facet dish to oblige any Chinese language-fashion number one dish. include eggplant and snow peas presented with an aspect of browned rice for an elegant weekday supper."

Ingredients

1 tbsp oil

1 lb zucchini reduce into 1/4 inch cuts half of container veggie lover stock

Two tsp mild soy sauce 1 tbsp dry sherry

One tsp broiled sesame oil

Instructions

Warm temperature an intensive work or overwhelming skillet over excessive warmth until the point while reasonably warm at that point include the oil. On the factor, while the oil is heated, encompass the zucchini and ginger. Panfry 1 minute. Consist of the soup, soy sauce, and sherry. Panfry over high warmth till the factor when the stock chefs down a bit and the zucchini are clean delicate. Expel from the heat, sprinkle with sesame oil and serve.

Sichuan Spicy Tangerine 'Chicken'

A wealthy, zesty and complex Szechwan-fashion(or Sichuan) dish served over a bed of crisp Chinese noodles, cellophane noodles or a thin egg noodle, as an example, vermicelli.

Ingredients

Three tbsp dry sherry

1 tbsp mild soy sauce

12 ounces company or extra company tofu, cut into half inch dice, or 2 glasses completed soy protein lumps or cutlets which have been reconstituted in veggie lover soup/stock and reduce into half of the inch portions

Half glass flour Sauce:

2 tbsp oil

Half tsp dried pink bean stew chips discretionary: 1/4 tsp Sichuan pepper

One loading tbsp newly ground tangerine or orange peel (orange component just, preferably herbal) 1 tbsp rice, juice or white wine vinegar

1 cup veggie lover soup

Hurl the sherry and soy sauce with the tofu and marinate for no less than ten mins. Hurl the marinated tofu inside the flour, saving the extra marinade.

Instructions

Warm temperature a great wok or overwhelming skillet over high warmth. At the factor, while it is warm, consist of 1 tbsp of the oil. On the point, while the oil is heated, encompass the half floured tofu 3-D squares. Panfry until the point that they're virtually sparkling and caramelized. Expel them from the skillet, cover the second tbsp of oil, let it heat and cook dinner the relaxation of the tofu in a similar way.

Consist of the fundamental institution of tofu lower back to the dish alongside the pepper chips, Sichuan pepper, and tangerine peel. Panfry for a second, at that factor, include the vinegar, remaining marinade and inventory. Cook over excessive warm temperature until the element that the massive majority of the stock dissipates. Serve hot.

Dan Dan Noodles

A Dan Dan Noodles recipe it attempted, actual, and genuine. With this method, you could attempt out this highly spiced, numbing Dan Dan Noodles Sichuan classic at domestic!

Ingredients

4oz thin rice noodles or 6 oz spaghettini or Japanese soba noodles or angel hair pasta 1 1/2 cups warm vegetarian broth

1 tbsp peanut butter Sauce:

1 tbsp oil

One medium onion, chopped

Four dried Chinese black mushrooms, soaked in hot water for 20 mins, stems discarded and sliced two cloves garlic, minced non-obligatory: 1 tbsp chopped Sichuan pickled vegetables

1/three cup soy protein granules soaked in 1/4 cup boiling water or half cup of vegetarian hamburger crumbles 1 tbsp light soy sauce

1 tbsp brown bean paste or mild miso 1 tbsp chili garlic paste

Half tbsp cornstarch mixed with 2 tbsp bloodless water 2 tbsp chopped green onion

1 tbsp roasted sesame oil

Boil the noodles in masses of water consistent with packet instructions. Drain in a colander. Blend the hot broth with the peanut butter. Hold heat.

Instructions

Heat a wok or heavy skillet over high heat. While it's warm, add the oil. When the oil is heated, then add up the onion, mushrooms and garlic and the pickled greens, if using. Stir-fry until the onions melt, adding a chunk of water as necessary to save you scorching. Add the textured soy protein, soy sauce, brown bean paste and chili paste. When it bubbles, stir in the cornstarch mixture and stir until thickened. Do away with from warmth.

Run warm water over the noodles, drain, and divide them among two heated soup bowls. Warmness the broth if essential and pour over the noodles. Divide the sauce evenly among the two pans, pinnacle with the chopped green onions and drizzle with the sesame oil. Serve straight away.

Gluten dough

Ingredients

1/2 containers pure gluten powder (organic wheat gluten) 2 mugs cold water cooking soup:

Four cups of water

6-inch piece kombu kelp 1/2 tbsp salt

Four dried Chinese dark mushrooms 2 tbsp lemon juice

1 tbsp sugar

One tsp dried garlic

Instructions

To influence the homemade gluten, to combine the gluten flour and the water. Blend until if frames a smooth, firm

Batter. Massage quickly. Keep your hands wet when dealing with the mixture of whatever remains of steps.

For "scallops": Shape the crude gluten mixture into a long move around 1 inch in the distance across. Cut into little adjusts like thin scallops. Blend the cooking soup fixings and heat to the point of boiling. Drop in the gluten changes and stew for 30 minutes. Refrigerate overnight in the cooking stock.

For "angle": level the crude gluten into thin "filet" shapes. If your pieces are too huge, simply cut them. Blend the cooking soup and convey to a low bubble. Include the gluten "filets" and come back to a low bubble, instead of a stew and cook for 30 minutes. It makes gentler seitan. Refrigerate overnight in the cooking juices.

For "mollusks": Tear the homemade gluten into modest bits. Heat the cooking stock to the point of boiling and drop in the gluten pieces. Bubble for 3 minutes and refrigerate overnight in the cooking soup.

For "shrimp": cut the raw gluten into little wedge shapes around 1/2 long and 1/2 inch thick. Blend the simmering stock and convey to a stew. Drop in the gluten and stew for 30 minutes. Refrigerate overnight in cooking soup.

Buddha's "Chicken"

It is a customary yuba (bean curd skin) formula utilized by Chinese Buddhist veggie lovers. It makes a delicious canapé. Remains can be hacked and used as a part of diminishing entirety stuffings or rice and noodle dishes. On the off chance that you use new yuba, which needs no dousing, this dish rushes to plan. It's anything but complicated to make whether you utilize new or dried yuba.

Ingredients

Three expansive sheets crisp yuba (bean curd skin) around 16 creeps in the distance across, cut down the middle, or 3 substantial rectangular sheets dried yuba

1/3 veggie lover soup

1/2 tbsp light soy sauce two tsp grungy sugar

1/2 tbsp broiled sesame oil for profound fricasseeing

Instructions

If utilizing the dried yuba, handle the sheets painstakingly and absorb warm water for 5 – 10 minutes. Pat them dry and cut down the middle.

Blend the soup, soy sauce, sugar and sesame oil in a little pot and warmth until the point when the sugar is broken up. Fill a bowl and permit to cool marginally.

Spread a 12x6 inch bit of fine cheesecloth or thin white cotton sheeting over a treated sheet. Place a half-sheet of the new or reconstituted dried yuba on the layer.

Brush the yuba with soy sauce blend. Cover with another bit of yuba and brush. Rehash until the more significant part of the yuba and sauce is spent. If there is some sauce left finished, pour it over the yuba and brush uniformly towards the edges.

Roll the piles of sheets into a minimal barrel and wrap it in the fabric. A tie closes with white string. Steam the roll, secured, over bubbling water for 10 minutes.

Evacuate painstakingly and cut the move into four segments, slantingly. Warmth the oil 350F in wok or skillet, or deep fryer. Drop in the steps, remaining back to abstain from splattering and profound broil until brilliant dark colored. It will take just a couple of moments. Deplete the moves on paper.

To serve, cut corner to corner into 1/2 inch adjusts and serve hot or frosty.

Chinese Style "Beefy" Seitan

This mixture of mushrooms, soy sauce, and crimson wine supply this seitan a deep umami flavor. Making your meat alternative may appear to be a complicated project, but this recipe is simple to follow and will go away you with outcomes ways better than processed, packaged seitan

Ingredients

cup bloodless water

tbsp darkish or mushroom soy sauce 2 tbsp ketchup

Two tsp Marmite, yeast extract or darkish miso, mixed with half cup hot water until dissolved 1/four tsp garlic granules

1/4 tsp onion powder

Two tsp Kitchen Bouquet or different gravy browner

One 1/four cups pure gluten powder (critical wheat gluten)

Additional ingredients: 1 tbsp light soy sauce 1 tbsp dry sherry

1 tbsp roasted sesame oil

Instructions

Mix the broth ingredients. In a small bowl, blend the gluten powder with 1 cup of the broth. Stir until a dough forms. Knead the dough a chunk to very well mix. Roll the dough right into a log and reduce it into 48 more or less equal-length slices or pieces.

Mix the final broth with half of the cup water and extra secret agent sauce and sherry in a medium saucepan. Convey to a boil. Drop in 12 pieces of gluten. Boil for four mins, then take away them with a slotted spoon and location in a bowl. Upload any other 1/2 cup water to the broth and bring to a boil once more, then drop 12 additional portions of gluten in and boil for four mins. Repeat this two greater instances till all the gluten cooked.

You can upload more than half of cup water the remaining time. Just make sure the gluten pieces are more significant or much less covered with the liquid while they prepare dinner.

When all of the gluten cooked, warmth the sesame oil in a big heavy skillet and upload the gluten portions together with the ultimate broth. Cowl and prepare dinner over medium-low heat for about 20 minutes till all the food is absorbed, and the gluten is firm. Stir because it cooks.

vicinity the gluten in a included field and refrigerate or freeze.

Asparagus Beef with Black Bean Sauce

Very good and less complicated than you anticipate. In case you substituted green beans and onions for the asparagus. You'll genuinely make this again. Speedy, easy, healthy and yummy.

Ingredients

Cooking sauce:

Half of cup cold water or mild vegetarian broth 1 tbsp sweet soy sauce

1 tbsp cornstarch

Half tsp mild unbleached sugar

2 cups Chinese fashion "Beefy" Seitan, cut into slivers two tsp dry sherry

One tsp water

One tsp cornstarch

One tsp mild soy sauce 1 tbsp oil

Two cloves garlic, minced or beaten

Two tsp fermented black beans, mashed with a fork

1 lb asparagus, and trimmed and cut diagonally into 1-inch portions 2 tbsp water

Instructions

Combine the cooking sauce elements in a bowl and set apart mix the seitan slivers with the sherry, one tsp water, one tsp cornstarch and one tsp soy sauce in a bowl.

Warm a considerable wok or heavy skillet over high heat. While it's miles hot, upload the oil. When the oil is heated, upload the garlic and fermented black beans. Stir-fry for some seconds then upload the marinated seitan. Stir-fry for three mins, then do away with to a bowl.

Upload the asparagus and onion to the pan, and stir-fry for 30 seconds. Add the 2 tbsp water to the pan, cowl and prepare dinner for two mins. Get rid of the duvet, upload the seitan aggregate and cooking sauce. Stir prepare dinner till the sauce has thickened. Serve right away with rice.

Onion-fragrant Red Lentils

This delicately hot dish utilizes a North Indian strategy called tadka or chaunk: seasonings are sizzled in hot oil or elucidated margarine, at that point twirled into the lentils just before serving for a considerable flavor help.

Ingredients

Three glasses of water (750ml) water

cup (250ml) red lentils

¼ tsp turmeric

½ tsp salt one tsp sugar

tbsp vegetable oil (utilize mustard oil on the off chance that you have it) 2 narrows clears out

Two entire red chilies

½ tsp kalonji seeds

cup (250ml) meagerly cut fragmented onion one little green bean stew, cleaved and seeded one tsp garam masala

tbsp crisp lime or lemon juice

1 tbsp finely cleaved crisp cilantro/coriander Method

Instructions

Get water to heat up a container over medium warmth. Include lentils. Include turmeric and stew, secured until the point when lentils are delicate, around 15 minutes. They should break with less effort when squeezed amongst thumb and pointer.

Include salt and sugar. Puree the blend in a blender until smooth. Come back to the dish and keep warm.

Then, warm oil in a skillet over medium-low warmth. Broil sound leaves and red chilies until the point that the chilies obscure. Include kalonji seeds and sear for a couple of moments. Broil the onion until luxuriously sautéed yet not consumed, 15 to 18 minutes, mixing continually. Mix in green bean stew. Pour this blend over the pureed lentils. Casserole for 2-3 minutes.

Expel from warm. Mix in garam masala, lime juice and cilantro. Topping with lemon wedges and

Tart Red Lentils

A sweet-smelling lentil tart in light of a straightforward blend of aromatics and broiled vegetables finished with a light sprinkling of Parmesan.

Ingredients

Three glasses (750ml) water

One glass (250ml) red lentils

1 tbsp peeled, minced crisp ginger

One tsp crisp green stew, seeded and cleaved

½ tsp salt one tsp sugar

½ tsp tamarind focus

One tsp vegetable oil (or mustard oil)

¼ tsp dark mustard seeds

½ tsp five-zest, broiled and ground
Method

Instructions

Get water to heat up a container over medium warmth. Include lentils. Include turmeric and stew, secured until the point when lentils are delicate, around 15 minutes. They should efficiently break when squeezed amongst thumb and pointer.

Puree this blend with the ginger and green stew in a blender until smooth. Come back to the dish and convey to stew. Include salt, sugar, and tamarind and mix to break down the tamarind. Expel from warm.

Then, warm oil in a 6-inch skillet over a medium-low warmth. Sear dark mustard seeds for a couple of moments. When the seeds begin popping, expel from mild and pour substance over lentil blend. Stew lentils 2 or 3 more minutes. Blend in 5 flavors. Cover and let remain for a couple of minutes to build up the characteristics. Enhance with lemon wedges and crisp cilantro.

Green split peas in zesty mustard sauce

When I required a snappy however fulfilling feast answer for end an unusually sad and attempting week. In the midst of misfortune, it's anything but complicated to turn to eatery dinners, yet I always remember that home-cooked suppers are all the more supporting, as well as less expensive and by and large unrivaled in taste. The fiery kick of this dish enjoyably adjusted by the quieted sweetness of the darker sugar.

Ingredients

Four mugs (1 liter) of water

One glass (250ml) green split peas one sound leaf

¼ tsp turmeric

½ tsp salt

1 ½ tbsp vegetable oil (or mustard oil) 1 tbsp peeled minced new ginger

One green bean stew seeded and hacked

Two tsp dark mustard seeds, ground to a powder, blended with four tsp water and permitted to remain for 30 minutes

3 tbsp dried destroyed or chipped sweetened coconut, ground in a blender to a coarse powder (or crisply ground or destroyed coconut blended with ½ tsp sugar.

Instructions

Convey water to bubble. Lower warm somewhat. Include split peas, sound leaf, and turmeric and stew secured until the point when peas are delicate, 40 – 45 minutes. Amid this period, reveal infrequently and blend, including a tbsp or so of boiling water I the blend adheres to the base of the skillet. Include salt. Keep warm.

In the interim, warm oil in a skillet over medium-low warmth. Broil ginger and green bean stew until the point when ginger gently cooked, 1-2 minutes. Include mustard glue and sear for one more moment, mixing every so often (you may need to keep the skillet incompletely secured for a couple of moments if the flavors begin to splatter the cooking territory). Include coconut and mix a few times. Expel from warm. Pour over the pea blend and mix. Cover and let remain for 15 minutes to build up the flavors. Trim with cilantro.

Down home chick pea stew

This down-home Chickpea Stew is a hearty and filling plant-based dish with the intention to hold you full and warm this wintry weather!

Ingredients

2 ½ tbsp vegetable oil (mustard oil favored) 1 bay leaf

2 ½ cups (625ml) finely chopped onion 1 tbsp minced garlic

1 tbsp peeled, minced ginger

½ tsp turmeric

Two tsp floor cumin

Two tsp ground coriander

One small fresh inexperienced chili, seeded and chopped

½ cup (125ml) chopped tomatoes

¼ tsp salt

1 ½ cups (375ml) cooked chickpeas or a 16oz (450g) can of chickpeas, drained garnish: slightly uncooked onion jewelry, chopped Roma tomatoes, freshly cut cilantro

Instructions

Warmness oil in a skillet over medium warmth. Add bay leaf and onion. Fry onion until richly browned however now not burnt, 15 –20 minutes, stirring often and reducing heat to medium-low halfway via cooking.

Stir in ginger and garlic and cook several mins. Upload turmeric, cumin, coriander and fresh chili and mix properly. Add tomatoes and salt. Lower warmth slightly, cover and cook dinner till tomatoes crumble and a thick sauce form, about 10 minutes. Stir on occasion to save you sticking, adding a tbsp of water is essential. Add chickpeas cover and prepare dinner for five extra minutes. Eliminate from heat and allow stand, included, for a few minutes to help broaden the flavors. Garnish with onion, tomatoes, and cilantro.

Serving piping hot.

Festive Chickpeas with coconut and whole spices

A customary clean coconut curry with chickpeas, roused by utilizing Indian flavors. This garbanzo bean curry skirts the mind-boggling steps, however, doesn't hold back on taste! Surely veggie lover and without gluten. Moreover liberated from grains, soy, and nuts.

Ingredients

One glass (250ml) chana dal (split chickpeas), absorbed a solitary day in five mugs (1 liter) of water

¼ tsp turmeric

One entire crisp green bean stew

½ tsp salt

One tsp ground cumin 2 tbsp raisins

1 ½ tbsp vegetable oil (mustard oil favored) 1 cove leaf

One whole dried purple bean stew

Five finish cardamom cases

2 inch (5cm) cinnamon stick two entire cloves

¼ tsp kalonji seeds

tbsp seeded, cleaved shimmering green bean stew

tbsp dried chipped or destroyed sweetened coconut (or crisply ground or destroyed coconut blended with one tsp sugar

¼ tsp garam masala

Instructions

Convey chana dal and the drenching water to bubble in a large container over medium warmth. Transfer turmeric and whole bean stew. Stew, covered, 60 minutes, or till the dal could be extraordinarily smooth and breaks easily while squeezed amongst thumb and forefinger. At some phase in this period, reveal and frequently mix, including 1-2 tbsp of water if the dal begins off evolved to glue to the base. Dispose of whole stew.

Include salt and cumin. Dispose of from warm.

Puree 1 container (250ml) of the dal mix in a blender, including a little water if basic. backpedal to the skillet. include raisins. convey to stew at that point keep warm.

Warmth oil in a dish over medium-low warmth. Sear sound leaf and red bean stew until the point when the stew obscures. Broil cardamom, cinnamon, and cloves for 5 seconds. Transfer kalonji and sear each other couple of moments. Flip warm to low. Include slashed green stew and coconut and cook supper for a couple of moments, blending continuously. Discard from mild. Transfer this zest total to the dal. Stew 2-3 additional mins. Expel dal from warm. Mix in garam masala. Trimming with lemon wedges, sprinkle with whole cilantro leaves and serve.

Fiery Potatoes

A suitable companion of mine would most likely be humiliated on the off chance that he realized that I'm disclosing to you he utilized the expressions of John Mellencamp to portray the warmth of these potatoes: "it harms so great." And so said companion might stay anonymous.

Ingredients

2 tbsp vegetable oil (mustard oil favored)

½ tsp dark mustard seeds

¼ tsp fenugreek seeds

1 tbsp peeled, minced crisp ginger one green stew seeded and slashed

¼ tsp turmeric

½ tsp salt

a dash of ground red bean stew or cayenne pepper (or to taste)

1 ½ lb (750g) cooked potatoes (around five medium) cut into 1-inch shapes (2.5 cm) at room temperature

¼ glass (60ml) dried chipped or destroyed sweetened coconut ground in a blender to a coarse powder or natural ground or destroyed coconut blended with ½ tsp sugar

1 tbsp finely cleaved new cilantro

Instructions

Warmth oil in a skillet over a medium-low warmth. Include mustard seeds. When the seeds begin popping include fenugreek, ginger and stew and turmeric, blending frequently. Keep the skillet halfway secured to keep the mustard seeds from flying out.

Include salt, red pepper and potatoes and broil for a moment or something like that, mixing continually. Swing warmth to low. Include coconut and cilantro and blend well. Expel from warm. Serve hot or at room temperature.

Spicy Home Fries

Who doesn't love domestic fries? This enticing heated variant is whatever but hard to make for any dinner of the day. There may be a little warmer temperature and a ton of get-up-and-move.

Ingredients

1 ½ lb (750g) unpeeled potatoes (round five medium) reduce into 1 inch (2.4 cm) 3D squares

Water for effervescent potatoes

½ tsp salt

2 ½ tbsp vegetable oil (mustard oil favored) 1 narrows leaf

One whole dried purple bean stew

½ tsp asafoetida powder one tsp sugar

1 tbsp ground cumin

a sprint of floor pink bean stew or cayenne (to taste)

½ tsp garam masala method

Instructions

Warmness up the potatoes with water to cowl and salt till the point when the vegetables are sensitive yet at the same time maintain their shape, 15-20 minutes. Dissipate. Permit cooling to room temperature.

Warmth 2 tbsp of the oil in a skillet over a medium warm temperature. Sear potatoes to the point that they flip medium darker, five-6 minutes, turning regularly. Evacuate with an opened spoon and placed aside.

Add ultimate ½ tbsp oil to a similar skillet and heat over medium-low warm temperature. Broil inlet leaf and pink stew until the factor while the bean stew obscures. Sprinkle asafoetida over the flavors. Encompass salt sugar potatoes cumin and crimson pepper. Sear for two-five mins to mix flavors, blending often. Expel from warm. Blend in garam masala. Serve hot or at room temperature.

Potatoes braised in rich tart sauce

The combination of potatoes, cheese, Francis Bacon and garlic dip in this recipe is terrific," says Leslie Cunnian of Peterborough, Ontario. "The skins can be served as an appetizer or as a side dish with a prime roast rib or any other entree you pick."

Ingredients

1 tbsp plus two tsp to 3 tbsp vegetable oil (mustard oil desired) 1 lb (1/2 kg) potatoes (approximately four medium) reduce into 1inch cubes two entire dried pink chilies

½ tsp asafoetida powder

3 tbsp peeled minced fresh ginger one inexperienced chili seeded and chopped two tsp ground cumin

A dash of red chili powder or cayenne (or to flavor)

½ tsp salt

½ tsp sugar

½ cup (125ml) water

1 tsp tamarind listen technique

Instructions

Warmth 2 tbsp oil in a skillet over medium warmness. Fry potatoes till they turn medium brown, 6 –7 mins, turning often. Do away with the slotted spoon and set apart.

Upload 1 tbsp oil to the skillet and heat over medium-low heat. Fry crimson chilies until they darken. Sprinkle asafoetida onto the chilies. Upload ginger, fresh chili, cumin, crimson pepper, salt and sugar and stir sometimes. Stir inside the potatoes. Add water and simmer, included until vegetables are soft but still preserve their form, 15 20 minutes.

Upload tamarind and stir gently to combine it with the potatoes. Dispose of from warmness and permit stand blanketed for ten mins to broaden the flavors. Garnish with cilantro to serve.

Potato skin fry

The blend of potatoes, cheddar, Francis Bacon and garlic plunge on this formula is top notch," says Leslie Cunnian of Peterborough, Ontario. "The skins might be filled in as a tidbit or as a perspective dish with high cook rib or some other course you pick."

Ingredients

1 tbsp besan (chickpea flour)

One container immovably pressed potato peels, lessen into 1 ½ inch (4cm) lengths 1 tbsp vegetable oil

1 tbsp white poppy seeds

½ tsp salt

Instructions

A run of ground pink stew or cayenne pepper (or to enhance) technique

Put besan in a paper sack and include the potato peels. Close the pack firmly and shake 8 – 10 cases till peels are pointlessly secured.

Warm oil in a non-stick skillet over the medium low fire. Include poppyseeds and sauté until delicately seared, a couple of moments. Transfer salt and purple pepper. Include the peels and broil until medium dark colored a crips, 10 – 15 mins, always mixing (the skins will splash up the oil quick yet keep up to sear them). Detract from warm. Serve warm or at room temperature.

Rich roasted eggplant

This broiled eggplant (otherwise known as aubergine) has a great creamy profound taste and a chewy, succulent surface.

Keep a tub or baggie in the refrigerator amid the late spring, and add a modest bunch to the side of a serving of mixed greens plate with a light sprinkle of ground parmesan on it — delectable.

Ingredients

medium eggplant, around 1 lb (½ kg)

tbsp vegetable oil (mustard oil favored)

¼ tsp kalonji seeds

1 to 2 entire green chilies

One glass (250ml) finely cleaved onion 1 tbsp minced garlic

1 tbsp peeled, minced crisp ginger

¼ tsp turmeric

½ tsp salt

½ tsp sugar

½ glass (125ml) cleaved tomatoes 1 tbsp finely slashed cilantro Method

Instructions

Preheat grill to 450F/230C gas check 8. Cut eggplant down the middle the long way and place on an un-lubed heating sheet with the chopping side down. Prepare for 30 to 40 minutes or until the point when the eggplant wrinkles and feels delicate to the touch when squeezed. The planning will change contingent upon the thickness of the eggplant.

Enable the eggplant to cool. Dispose of the skin, finely slash the fragile living creature and crush it with a fork.

Warmth oil in a skillet over medium-low warmth. Broil kalonji seeds and whole chilies for a couple of moments. Include onion and sear until the point that it is luxuriously cooked yet not consumed, 8 – 10 minutes. Include garlic and ginger and mix a few times. Include hacked green bean stew, turmeric, salt, sugar, and tomatoes. Stew, secured, until the point when tomatoes have broken down into a sauce, around 10 minutes. Dispose of whole chilies, if wanted.

Include the eggplant and stew, secured, 10 minutes to mix flavors, mixing incidentally to forestall staying. Expel from warm. Let stand obtained for 15 minutes to help build up the flavors. Include cilantro and blend well. Enhancement of green onion and serve.

Butternut Squash in Mustard Sauce

Lay up squash or pumpkin with a creamy, creamy sauce and bubbling melted cheese to make this indulgent side dish - serve with a Sunday roast or sausages

Ingredients

2 tbsp vegetable oil (mustard oil preferred)

One bay leaf

One whole dried red chili

¼ tsp kalonji seeds

One green chili seeded and chopped

¼ tsp turmeric

4 cups (1 liter) butternut squash cut into 1-inch (2.5 cm) cubes

½ tsp salt

½ tsp sugar

¼ cup (60ml) water

One tsp black mustard seeds ground to a powder, mixed with two tsp water and allowed to stand for 30 minutes

¼ cup dried flaked or shredded sweetened coconut or freshly grated or shredded coconut mixed with ½ tsp sugar

Instructions

Heat the oil over the medium level of low heat in a skillet. Fry the bay leaf, and the red chili until the chili blackens. Fry kalonji seeds for a few seconds. Add green chili and turmeric and stir a few times. Stir in butternut squash, salt, sugar, and water.

Simmer covered, 10 minutes. Add mustard paste and stir gently to mix with sauce. Simmer, covered, until the vegetables are tender but not mushy, 5 – 13 minutes. Carefully stir in coconut. Remove from heat. Scatter cilantro on top and serve.

Cabbage Potato Extravaganza

This utterly scrumptious, elegant vegetable element dish of Parmesan Roasted Cabbage Wedges befell from cleaning out our refrigerator. The result is a plate desirable for your lovely dinner party

Ingredients

2 ½ tbsp mustard oil

¾ lb (375g) peeled potatoes lessen into 1 inch (2.5cm) cubes

½ tsp cumin seeds

6 cups (1 liter 500ml) finely shredded cabbage one green chili seeded and chopped

¼ cup plus 2 tbsp water

¾ tsp salt

½ tsp turmeric one ¼ tsp sugar

a dash of red chili powder or cayenne pepper (or to taste)

½ cup (125ml) thawed frozen peas

½ tsp garam masala

Instructions

Heat 2 tbsp oil in a 12 inch, deep-sided pan or Dutch oven over medium heat. Add potatoes and fry till medium brown, 5-8 mins, stirring frequently. Remove with a slotted spoon and set apart.

Add the closing ½ tbsp oil to the pan and warmth over medium-low warmness. Add cumin seeds and fry for some seconds until lightly browned. Add cabbage, green chili and ¼ cup (60ml) water. Lower temperature slightly and prepare dinner exposed till cabbage is limp, 6-8 mins, stirring regularly. Stir in salt, turmeric, sugar, pink pepper, 2 tbsp water and the potatoes.

Simmer, covered, till potatoes are gentle, 18-20 mins, adding peas during the last 2-3 mins. Put off by warmness and mix in garam masala. Permit stand for a few minutes to help expand the flavors.

Steamed Spicy Cauliflower

This superhealthy curry aspect dish is a Punjabi staple. Deliciously spicy, it is also an excellent source of vitamin C

Ingredients

1 tbsp ground cumin

1 tbsp ground coriander 2 tbsp water

1 ½ tsp sugar

¾ tsp salt

1 tbsp peeled clean ginger, grated one green chili seeded and chopped 2 tbsp mustard oil

four cups (1 liter) cauliflower reduce into florets 1 ½ inch (4cm) in diameter

½ lb (1/4kg) peeled potatoes (about 2 medium) reduce into 1 inch (2.5cm) cubes 1 cup (250ml) chopped tomatoes

¼ cup (60ml) water one bay leaf

Instructions

Integrate cumin and coriander with 2 tbsp water in a small bowl. Upload sugar salt, ginger, and green chili. Add oil and mix well.

Integrate cauliflower, potatoes, and tomatoes in a large bowl. Pour the spice mixture over the veggies and blend very well.

Warm the water in a non-stick skillet as a minimum 10 inches (25cm) in diameter. As quickly as it comes to a boil, upload bay leaf, and the vegetable mixture. You do not want to stir it. Simmer, tightly blanketed, until the

potatoes are tender and cauliflower is still slightly crunchy 15-20 minutes. Garnish with cilantro and serve.

Cauliflower and Potatoes in Roasted Red Chilli Sauce

I made this Recipe, and this was top and smooth to make. It turned into a pleasant alternative. I suppose your kids would favor it a piece more with a cheese sauce on pinnacle

Ingredients

1 ½ tbsp plus two tsp of a few ½ tbsp vegetable oil (mustard oil preferred)

1 lb (½ kg) peeled potatoes (approximately 3 medium) cut into 1-inch (2.5cm) cubes 1 tsp sugar

1 bay leaf

¼ tsp black mustard seeds

½ tsp cumin seeds

¼ tsp turmeric

1 tbsp peeled, clean ginger, grated 3 cloves garlic, beaten.

½ cup (125ml) chopped tomatoes

½ tsp salt

¾ cup (175ml) water to two tsp purple chilli paste*(recipe under) 2 tsp ground cumin tsp floor coriander cups cauliflower reduce into florets 1 ¾ inches (four.5cm) in diameter

¼ cup thawed frozen peas

¼ tsp garam masala tbsp fresh lemon juice

Instructions

Warmness 2 tbsp oil in a large skillet over medium warmth. Fry potatoes till they turn medium brown, approximately five mins, turning often. Remove with a slotted spoon and set apart.

Add the final 1-½ tbsp oil to the skillet and heat over medium-low warmness. Add sugar and stir till it turns barely brown. Fry bay leaf, black mustard seeds, and cumin seeds till they begin to crackle. Add turmeric, ginger, and garlic and stir several instances. Add tomatoes, salt, and water. Add potatoes, crimson chili

paste, floor cumin, and coriander. Simmer, included, for 10 minutes.

Add cauliflower and simmer, included, until each cauliflower and potatoes accomplished, some other 10-15 minutes: the cauliflower must be crisp-soft. Add peas and simmer, blanketed, one more minute. Put off from warmth. Blend in garam masala. Permit stand covered for a couple of minutes to help increase the flavors.

Sprinkle lemon juice and cilantro on the pinnacle and serve.

Purple chili paste:

Dried purple chili, made right into a paste, adds a rich, warm flavor and sweet hotness to a dish. You may roast the chilies first also to beautify the sauce. Put 2 to 4 whole dried red chilies on an ungreased griddle or skillet over a low warmth. Flip as quickly as they start to darken on the bottom. Repeat for the alternative facet. Soak the chilies (roasted or no longer) in warm water for approximately 15 minutes or till they may be tender. You could get rid of the seeds to reduce the hotness or leave them in if they may be moderate. Grind the flesh with a mortar and pestle or in a mini-chopper using two tsp or so of the soaking water.

Do no longer substitute commercial crimson chili paste, available in Asian markets. This paste consists of other elements and could modify the flavor of a dish.

Spicy Stuffed Tomatoes

Kick off your subsequent party the right manner and serve those baked tomatoes stuffed with a creamy filling made from sour cream, Sargento® Shredded Sharp Cheddar Cheese - first-rate cut, spices, and minced garlic. Serve with crunchy breadsticks for best snacking.

Ingredients

Two tbsp vegetable oil

¼ tsp asafoetida powder

¾ cup (175ml) of finely chopped onion 1 tbsp peeled minced fresh ginger

One inexperienced chili seeded and chopped

¼ tsp turmeric

2 tbsp besan (chickpea flour)

¼ tsp salt

1 tbsp finely chopped cilantro method

Instructions

Do away with the dark stem give up from 8 of the tomatoes. Cautiously hole out each plant by using getting rid of the pulp and seeds; discard the seeds but save the flesh. Chop enough of the remaining two tomatoes, discarding the seeds, to make a ¼ cup (60ml) collectively with the reserved pulp. Set apart.

Warmth oil in a skillet over medium-low warmth. Sprinkle asafoetida over the oil. Fry onion till it is richly browned however not burnt, eight −10 minutes, stirring continuously. Upload ginger, fresh chili and turmeric and stir sometimes. Stir within the besan. Decrease the heat slightly. Upload the reserved tomato pulp, salt, and cilantro.

Prepare dinner until the pulp disintegrates into the sauce, about 2 minutes, stirring frequently. Transfer to a bowl and allow cool slightly.

Stuff the hollowed tomatoes with this aggregate and place upright in a baking pan. If they will now not stand because of their point ends, area a crumpled piece of aluminum foil on the lowest of the cooking container and make small hollows in the foil to aid the tomatoes upright. Or you can use a muffin pan.

Just earlier than serving, preheat oven to 400F / 200C / fuel mark 6. Bake the tomatoes till they may be gentle but hold their color and form, 7- 12 mins (the timing will vary with the firmness and size of the tomatoes. Do now not over bake or the tomatoes will darken and their skin will wrinkle. Serve right away.

Pureed greens with chilli and coconut over rice

Green curry with chunks of her thigh, infant spinach cashews, and fresh onions served over steamed rice with cilantro.

Ingredients

Five ½ cups (1 liter 375ml) firmly packed slivered greens (mustard veggies, collards, kale, fresh spinach). 1 tbsp mustard oil

Two tsp black mustard seeds, ground to a powder, blended with two tsp water and allowed to stand for 30 minutes

One green chili seeded and chopped.

¼ tsp of salt

2 tbsp of dried flaked or shredded sweetened coconut or freshly grated or shredded coconut combined with ¼ tsp sugar pure boiled rice

Instructions

Convey three-four tbsp water to a boil in a vast, deep sided pan. Upload the slivered greens. Cover and flip warmth to medium-low, and steam till the veggies are gentle but still maintain their color, four-5 mins. If using spinach, you want most effective a minute or.

To puree the vegetables: try this in batches: area about 2 tbsp water and approximately 2 cups of cooked greens in a blender. Don't use any more water than necessary to achieve a smooth puree.

Place the pureed greens in a sieve about 5 inches (2.5cm) in diameter. Rest the strainer over a tall tumbler to seize drippings. With the back of a large spoon, you must press down on the vegetables to squeeze out moisture. A cup of liquid should release into the tumbler. While no greater moisture comes out, set the greens aside.

Heat the oil in a skillet over medium-low warmness. Add mustard paste and green chili and stir a few times, retaining the skillet in part included if the mustard paste starts off evolved to splatter. Upload the greens and salt and stir a few times. Add coconut and blend properly. Dispose of from warmth. Serve about 2 tbsp per man or woman on top of boiled rice.

Vegetable Pullao

Create consolation in a pot with this beautiful melange. A simple, fast and satisfying rice meal made with the goodness of fresh garden vegetables.

Ingredients

Vegetable oil

¾ cup (175ml) carrots cut into ¾ inch (2cm) cubes

1 cup (250ml) cauliflower cut into florets 1 inch (2.5cm) in diameter

¼ cup (60ml) inexperienced beans reduce crosswise into ½ inch (1cm) pieces one bay leaf

6-eight cardamom pods

2-inch (5cm) cinnamon stick two entire cloves

1 cup (250ml) of finely chopped onion 1 tbsp peeled minced fresh ginger

One inexperienced chili seeded and chopped 2 tbsp unsalted raw cashews

1 tbsp raisins (ideally golden)

One ¼ cup (300ml) basmati or long grain white rice

¾ cup (175ml) chopped tomatoes

½ tsp salt

½ tsp sugar

½ to one tsp saffron, ground to a powder and soaked in 1 tbsp heat water for half-hour 2 cups (500ml) warm water

¼ cup (60ml) frozen peas, thawed

Instructions

Warmness 1 ½ tbsp oil in a pan over medium warmth. Fry carrots, cauliflower, and green beans until the vegetables gently browned three-5 minutes. Dispose of with a slotted spoon and set apart.

Add 2 ½ tbsp oil to the pan and warmth over medium-low heat. Upload bay leaf, cardamom, cinnamon and cloves and fry for some seconds. Upload onion and fry until translucent, about 2 minutes, stirring constantly. Add ginger, green chili, cashews and raisins and cook for a minute or so, stirring continuously.

Add rice and fry until opaque, three or so mins, stirring continuously. Upload tomatoes, salt, and sugar. The mixture of saffron and the soaking liquid. Upload hot water and convey to boil. Lower the heat slightly and simmer, protected, till a maximum of the water is absorbed and rice is tender about 12 minutes.

Vicinity veggies on the pinnacle of rice; do no longer stir. Simmer, included until rice is carried out, and greens are soft but the company, 5-10 mins. Vicinity peas on top of rice at some point of final 2 minutes of cooking. Remove from heat. Permit stand protected for 10 minutes to permit rice to grow to be plumper and fluffier. Serve garnished with brown-fried onions.

Puffed bread

Lavaş, now and then known as "balloon bread," is skinny and crispy and puffs up high as it cooks. It's served piping warm, with a hole middle complete of steam, as an appetizer before kebab food. You will regularly locate it observed via Turkish Tulum goat cheese, chunks of unsalted village butter, and a highly spiced tomato and pepper overwhelm known.

Ingredients

1 cup plus 1 tbsp (265ml) all reason flour 1 tsp baking powder

1 tbsp vegetable oil 6 tbsp heat water

extra flour for dusting vegetable oil for the in-depth frying approach

Instructions

Sift flour and baking powder right into a bowl. Make a well inside the middle, add oil and blend with your fingers until the aggregate resembles coarse crumbs. step by step upload water to shape a dough that holds collectively.

Knead and allow relaxation at room temperature for as a minimum half-hour.

Pinch off a part of the dough and make a ball about one ¾ inch (4cm) in diameter by way of rolling between the fingers of your palms. On the lightly floured work surface, you can roll out right into a disc approximately 4 ½ inches (11cm) in diameter and 1/16 inch (1.5mm) thick; if rolled too thin, it may not puff up. Shake off extra flour.

Warmness oil in a deep fat fryer or saucepan to 375F (190C). Cautiously drop a disc into the new oil. It's going to upward push to the surface and blow own trumpet without delay, either entirely or in numerous locations. Get rid of with a slotted spatula and drain on paper towels. For the reason that prepares dinner in some seconds, I fry one lunch at a time.

Coconut Scented Rice Pudding

This recipe is completely vegan and delicious (just motive it's vegan doesn't suggest it's now not scrumptious!). It has a mellowness from the coconut milk and a tartness from the orange juice flavor. It's additionally healthful for you.

Ingredients

¾ cup (175ml) basmati rice or different lengthy grain white rice 1 ½ cups (375ml) water

1 tbsp raisins (ideally golden)

2 tbsp toasted cashews or slivered almonds one tsp floor cardamom

¼ cup plus 1 tbsp (75ml) sugar

One ¼ cups (300ml) clean or unsweetened canned coconut milk approach

Instructions

Convey rice and water to boil in a pan. Simmer, included, until all of the water is absorbed and rice is gentle, 20 or so minutes.

Upload raisins, cashews, and cardamom. Dissolve sugar in the coconut milk and stir into the rice aggregate gently, that allows you to destroy the rice kernels no longer. Boost warmth slightly and cook dinner uncovered until the total thickens, 5 to ten minutes. do away with from heat. Allow cool barely. Garnish with pistachios and serve.

Poppy seed Sauce

A colorful but straightforward traybake for two- the creamy, vivid orange sauce lifts the dish with citrus and paprika flavors

Ingredients

One medium eggplant, approximately 1lb 2 tbsp vegetable oil

Two entire dried purple chiles 1/four tsp fenugreek seeds one half of tbsp minced garlic

One tsp seeded, chopped sparkling green chili 1/4 tsp turmeric

1/four cup water

2 tbsp white poppy seeds made right into a paste (toast the seeds in a dry skillet after which pulverize them in a mortar and pestle with a little water to make a dough)

Half tsp salt

1/2 tsp sugar

Instructions

Smoke and roast the eggplant: Preheat oven to 450F (230C). Cut eggplant in 1/2 lengthwise and location on an ungreased baking sheet with the reduce aspect down. Bake for 30 to 34 mins or till the eggplant wrinkles and feels tender to touch when pressed. Slice. Set aside.

Heat oil in a skillet over medium-low warmness. Fry red chilies until they darken. Add fenugreek, garlic and green chili and stir till garlic turns mild brown. Upload turmeric and water and bring to boil. Decrease the warmth barely and awaken within the eggplant slices. Add poppyseed paste, salt, and sugar and mix properly. Simmer included for 20 minutes, stirring once in a while to prevent sticking. Do away with from warmness. Let stand protected for a couple of minutes to develop flavors. Garnish with green onions.

Crisp Fried Eggplant

A delicious sauce that can serve without delay; at the pinnacle of the cooked broccoli or cauliflower, or chilled it and used it as a vegetable dip. The best way my children will consume broccoli or cauliflower!

Ingredients

1 cup besan (chickpea flour)

Half of tsp baking powder two tsp floor cumin 1/four tsp salt

1/2 tsp sugar

Two tsp vegetable oil

Half of cup undeniable soy yogurt 1 cup water

One small eggplant, up to 1lb, reduce into two half x 1/2 x 1/four inch portions vegetable oil for frying (as a minimum 2 inches deep)

Instructions

In a bowl, integrate besan, baking powder, cumin, salt, and sugar. Blend in oil and soy yogurt. Progressively add water, stirring with a spoon so that a clean batter bureaucracy. Some portions of eggplant in the batter. Get rid of with a slotted spoon.

Heat oil in a saucepan or deep fats fryer to 375F (190C). Heat oven to 200F (110C). Fry a few eggplant and slices at the same time until they flip golden brown all over, about a minute on each side, turning once. (cut one fried piece in half to peer if the inner appropriately cooked). Drain on paper towels. Serve straight away or maintain warm in the oven till all had fried.

Sweet and Tart Pumpkin

Do not just use pumpkin for savory dishes - its herbal sweetness makes it a brilliant base for desserts as correctly.

Ingredients

1 tbsp vegetable oil (mustard oil preferred) half of tsp asafoetida powder

1/four tsp kalonji seeds 1/2 tsp turmeric

One tsp seeded, chopped, sparkling inexperienced chili three/four tsp salt

three 1/2 sugar 3/four cup water

five cups peeled the sparkling pumpkin, or butternut squash reduce into 1/2 inch cubes

One 1/four tsp tamarind concentrate

Instructions

Warmth oil in a skillet over medium-low warmness. Sprinkle asafoetida over the oil. Add kalonji and fry for a few seconds. Upload turmeric, green chili, salt, and sugar. Upload water and pumpkin. Simmer, included, until veggies are tender but not mushy, 18 – 25 minutes.

Stir in tamarind lightly in order not to break the squash cubes. Cook dinner exposed for a minute or to be able to allow the sauce to thicken. If the sauce remains a little watery, mash a few of the vegetable cubes with the back or a spoon and mix in with the sauce. Cast off from warmth. Allow stand covered for a few minutes to help increase the flavors. Scatter cilantro on top.

Peanut Topped Greens

Thick, creamy, and full of flavor, these fresh beans and potatoes are served in a peanut sauce with a hint of Asian taste. The sauce made from creamy peanut butter combined with sesame oil and sweet chili oil, then crowned with chopped peanuts for additional crunch. The potatoes are tender and smooth, the beans are soft-crisp, and the dish is perfect served over a bed of quinoa.

Ingredients

6 cups firmly packed coarsely chopped hearty greens which includes sparkling spinach, chard, collard, kale and mustard vegetables

2 tbsp vegetable oil (mustard oil favored) 1 bay leaf

One complete dried crimson chili

1/4 tsp asafoetida powder

1 tsp seeded, chopped clean, green chili 1 tbsp peeled minced fresh ginger

1/4 tsp turmeric

1/8 tsp black pepper two tsp ground cumin 1/four tsp salt

Half of the cup soymilk

1/four unsalted dry roasted peanuts, coarsely chopped

Instructions

Steam the veggies until smooth and puree in a blender. Set apart.

Warmth oil in a heavy skillet over medium-low heat. Fry bay leaf and pink chili till the chili darkens. Sprinkle asafoetida on the pinnacle of purple chili. Stir in fresh chili, ginger, turmeric, black pepper, cumin, and salt. Add soymilk and cook till decreased to approximately half its extent, three – 5 minutes, stirring regularly.

Upload the pureed veggies. Cover and place over low warmness for 3-5 mins to blend the flavors and warmth the combination. Eliminate from warmness. Sprinkle peanuts on the pinnacle.

Lime Splashed Butternut Squash over Rice

This coconut lime butternut squash fried rice it just superb as an aspect dish served with your favored protein, like tofu, eggs or grilled chicken!

Ingredients

1 tbsp mustard oil (or vegetable oil) 1/2 tsp black mustard seeds

One tsp seeded, chopped fresh inexperienced chili (or to taste) half of tsp turmeric

2 cups mashed, cooked butternut squash half tsp salt

Three tbsp clean lime or lemon juice undeniable boiled rice

Instructions

Warmth oil in a skillet over medium-low warmth and fry the black mustard seeds. As quickly as the seeds begin popping, add green chili and turmeric and stir a few times. Add squash and salt.

Fry for two mins, stirring often. Eliminate from heat. Blend in lime juice. Serve a small amount of pure boiled rice garnished with fresh chili.

Coconut and Cilantro Chutney

This condiment, vivid in color and flavor, takes just minutes to make. It combines sweet coconut, peppery cilantro, and a piece of chile warmness to create a chutney worthy of pairing

Ingredients

Half of the cup water

2 tbsp sparkling lemon juice

1 cup dried flaked or shredded sweetened coconut

1/three cup firmly packed, coarsely chopped fresh cilantro (coriander) leaves 1 tbsp peeled coarsely chopped fresh ginger

1/2 tsp seeded coarsely chopped clean inexperienced chili (or to flavor) 1 tsp ground cumin

1/4 tsp salt

One tsp vegetable oil (mustard oil favored) half of tsp black mustard seeds

Instructions

Area water, lemon juice, coconut, cilantro, ginger, green chili, cumin and salt within the order given inside the field of a blender. Mixture until decreased to a thick puree, including a little extra water is necessary. Pour right into a small bowl.

Warmth oil in 6-inch skillet over medium-low warmth. Upload black mustard seeds. When the seeds start crackling, remove from heat. Upload to the contents of the bowl.

Hot and Spicy Bean Curd Burritos

Tofu has a custard-like texture and is to have in soft, firm and extra-firm types; the company is ultimate right here. Serve these hearty burritos crowned with purchased salsa and a few simple nonfat yogurt.

Ingredients

Olive oil

1lb greater company bean curd, drained and cut into 1/2 inch cubes two carrots, peeled and reduce into half of the inch chunks

One bunch broccoli, florets reserved and stalks reduce into half-inch chunks one pink bell pepper, cored and cut into half of the inch portions

One yellow bell pepper, cored and reduce into 1/2 inch portions two garlic cloves thinly sliced

Two medium crimson onions, diced salt, and pepper

Eight to 10 10-inch flour tortillas

Instructions

Warm several tbsp of olive oil in a large sauté pan or wok. Upload the bean curd and stir well to coat with oil. Sauté often stirring for 7 to ten mins or until the bean curd is brown on all aspects.

Add the carrots, and broccoli stalks stir nicely and sauté for 3-five mins stirring regularly. Stir in peppers, garlic, and onion and sauté for 3-5 minutes stirring frequently.

Cut the broccoli florets into little pieces and stir into the bean curd combination. Sauté for two-4 minutes, stirring often, the burrito submitting is carried out with the broccoli florets darken but are still crispy. Season to flavor with salt and pepper.

Positioned tortilla on a plate. Place several tbsp of filling at the tortilla. However, some salsa on top, roll up and serve.

Biker Beerittos

Ingredients

2 tbsp olive oil

2 tbsp chopped garlic two medium onions diced

Two clean cherry peppers minced

1 (19oz) can big crimson kidney beans, tired 1 tbsp liquid smoke

Half of tsp black pepper half tsp salt

Half of tsp ground cumin

One yellow bell pepper wire and reduce into strips one ripe beefsteak tomato, pureed

1 tbsp darkish molasses

1 (12oz) bottle of dark beer eight to 10 10-inch flour tortillas salsa

Instructions

Warm the olive oil in a heavy sauté pan over excessive heat. Add the garlic, onions and cherry peppers, stir to coat with oil and sauté for 3-5 minutes or until the onions are brown. Add the beans liquid smoke, black pepper, salt, and cumin. Reduce the warmth to medium, stir adequately and simmer for 10 minutes or until the liquid is absorbed.

Add the bell pepper and tomato puree stir well and simmer for 8 to 10 minutes or until the liquid is absorbed. Lessen the heat to low upload the molasses and beer and simmer for 8-10 minutes or until the sauce is decreased to a thick and creamy consistency.

Put tortilla on a plate.

Conventional flour tortillas - self-made and lots better than keeping offering. Do now not alternative vegetable oil or shortening for the lard.

Ingredients

Location numerous tbsp of filling at the tortilla, however a few salsa on the pinnacle, roll up and serve Black Eyed Soup

Three tbsp margarine

Two medium onions minced

1 sparkling lengthy narrow pink cayenne pepper, diced 1 (15oz) can black-eyed peas, rinsed

Two carrots cut into 1/four inch slices half of tsp salt

1/four tsp black pepper one tsp dried parsley 1/8 tsp celery seeds

1.5 cups cool water 1/8 tsp floor cumin

Instructions

In a cast iron skillet, soften 2 tbsp of margarine over medium warmness. Upload the onions and cayenne pepper and sauté 3-five minutes or until the onions are golden brown.

Location the black-eyed peas carrots salt black pepper parsley and celery seeds in a 2-quart saucepan and cowl with water. Convey to a boil. Add the sautéed onions and cayenne pepper, reduce heat to low and simmer for 30 to 40 minutes. Stir regularly to save you the peas from sticking to the bottom of the pot.

Do away with the soup from the warmth and allow to chill. Puree in a food processor or blender with the last 1 tbsp margarine and the cumin. Go back to the saucepan, reheat and serve.

Mean Black Bean Soup

Black bean soup is simple, clean, and just downright delicious. Frequently I'm going for the black bean soup for the toppings. I imply. C'mon. Avocado, tomato, sour cream, cilantro, cheese, a few extra cheese, jalapeño, and a little greater cheese. You guys load up your black bean soup too proper? If no longer I assume you're missing out on the splendor of this dish.

Ingredients

One anchor pepper stemmed seeded and torn into small portions one dried long narrow cayenne pepper, stemmed and beaten 1/4 cup boiling water

2 tbsp olive oil

One medium onion minced one carrot minced

One celery stalk minced

Half of the cup peeled whole tomatoes with their juice 1/2 tsp black pepper

1/4 tsp dried oregano one tsp salt

1/four tsp floor cumin

1 (19oz) can black beans

1 (12oz) bottle stout or dark beer

Instructions

The anchor and cayenne peppers in a small bowl. Cover with the boiling water and set apart to cool.

Warmness the oil in a large soup pot over medium heat. Upload the onion, carrot, and celery, stir nicely to coat with oil and sauté for 2-3 minutes or until the onion is transparent.

At the same time as the onion is sautéing, puree the re-hydrated peppers alongside the tomatoes in a blender for 1 minute, till comfortable and free of chunks. Add the puree and the final ingredients to the pot, bring the soup to the boil, then lessen the warmth to low. Cowl and simmer for 30 minutes stirring often to save you the beans from sticking to the lowest of the pot.

The use of a slotted spoon, remove 1 cup of the beans and set aside. Puree the relaxation of the soup in the blender or a meals processor. Return the puree and the reserved beans to the pot and reheat over the bottom viable warmness. Stir properly before serving.

Angel Pasta

If you are looking for a meal for two that would be perfect for a Valentine's Day meal, an anniversary dinner, or just a quick and easy supper on a busy day, you can't go wrong with this recipe from Tonya. It will fit just about any occasion, and it is incredibly fast and easy. And keep in mind that the recipe can be doubled or tripled for a larger family meal or dinner party.

Ingredients

14 sun-dried tomatoes, thinly sliced 7 tsp chopped garlic

2 dried long slim cayenne peppers, stemmed and crushed

1 ancho pepper, stemmed, seeded and torn into small pieces 1 cup boiling water

12 scallions

1/2 cup olive oil

lb angel hair pasta

Instructions

Fill a large pot with water and bring to a boil to cook the pasta.

Combine the sun-dried tomatoes, garlic and cayenne and ancho peppers in a small bowl and cover with the boiling water. Set aside and allow to cool to room temperature.

Trim the scallions. Remove the dark green tops and set aside. Cut the white and light green sections into 1/4-inch slices.

In a medium sauté pan, heat the olive oil over medium heat. Add the white and light green scallions and sauté for 3 to 5 minutes or until the scallions are golden brown. Add the pepper and sun-dried tomato mixture and stir well to deglaze the pan. Bring to a boil, reduce the heat and simmer for 15 minutes.

Remove the pan from the heat and mash the sauce well with a potato masher. Return to very low heat to keep warm while you prepare the pasta.

Cut the dark green scallion tops into 1/4 inch slices and set aside.

Cook the angel hair al dente, according to the package directions. Drain well, rinse to remove starch, and drain again. Toss with the sauce, garnish with the scallion tops and serve immediately.

Hot Nutty Noodles

Refrigerate any leftovers. To make the aggregate creamy once more, upload a spoonful or two of boiling water, and toss.

Ingredients

Six scallions

1/four cup peanut oil

2 sparkling lengthy slim crimson cayenne peppers, stemmed and minced one sparkling pink jalapeno pepper, stemmed and minced

Seven garlic cloves minced

1/2 cup unsalted roasted cashews, coarsely chopped 2 tbsp sesame seeds

1/2 cup chunky peanut butter 1 cup coconut milk

1/4 cup water

salt and pepper to taste 1 lb angel hair pasta

Instructions

Fill a huge pot with water and convey to a boil to cook dinner the pasta.

Trim the scallions. Do away with the dark inexperienced tops, reduce into 1/4 inch-thick slices and set apart. Mince the white and mild unskilled sections.

In a small pan or saucepan, warm the peanut oil over a low warm. Add the minced scallions, peppers and the garlic, the cashews and sesame seeds and sauté for three-five minutes or until the scallions are golden browns, being very careful no longer to burn the cashews and sesame seeds. Upload the peanut butter and stir until melted. Upload the coconut milk and stir nicely to blend. Slowly add the water, stirring continuously until nicely blended. Season with salt and pepper to flavor.

hold the sauté warm over very low warmth while you prepare the pasta, frequently stirring, so it does not separate. Cook the angel hair as in step with package deal instructions.

Just earlier than serving, add the darkish new pieces of scallion to the sauce and stir nicely. Drain the pasta carefully and toss with the sauce. Serve right now.

Smoky Bean Curd Stir Fry

All in all, this isn't only a pleasant dish to eat. However, it is straightforward to cook, requiring very few substances, most of them with ease to have in neighborhood Asian markets and your grocery shop. I noticeably propose, however, which you go out of your manner to pick out up a few sincerely correctly, thick sliced Sir Francis Bacon, no longer the skinny stuff from Oscar Mayer. If you are going to eat this a whole lot beef fat, allow or not it's the high-quality red meat fat you could locate.

Ingredients

1 (three.75 ounce) bag bean thread (cellophane) noodles 1 to 2 big broccoli stalks Seven scallions peanut or olive oil

2 or higher sparkling Serrano peppers stemmed and thinly sliced 6 or greater garlic cloves coarsely chopped

1-inch dice fresh ginger peeled and minced

Four carrots peeled and reduce into abnormal fashioned portions three celery stalks sliced three/four inches thick on a bias

1lb extra firm bean curd drained liquid smoke

One small zucchini quartered lengthwise and reduced into 1/four inch slices 1 cup snow peas, trimmed

1 (15oz) can baby corn, tired

Cut one red bell pepper cored into 3/4 inch squares salt and pepper

Instructions

Took a large pot of water to a boil. Upload the bean threads, stir, then cast off from heat and set aside to soak; they ought to be ready while the stir-fry is completed (if the package deal directions are one-of-a-kind, observe them).

Trim the broccoli, casting off the florets and breaking them into chunk-size portions; set aside. Cut the stalks into irregular chunks. Trim the scallions. Eliminate the darkish new tops and set aside. Cut the white and mild inexperienced sections into 3/4 inch-thick slices. Thinly slice the dark naive parts.

Heat numerous tbsp of oil in an entirely large sauté pan or wok. (it could be necessary to add higher as you add more ingredients). Positioned the Serrano peppers, garlic and ginger into sauté pan or wok. Stir-fry for 1 minute. Add the broccoli stalk and carrots and stir well to coat with oil. Stir-fry for 3 minutes. Upload the white and light inexperienced sections of the scallions along with the celery to the sauté pan or wok and stir-fry for two mins.

Area of the bean curd on a slicing board with the broad side up. Cut on diagonals into four triangles, then square each triangle piece on its longest side and cut in 1/2 from the tip toward the longest side. Slice every triangle chink into four slices. Area the bean curd pieces inside the warm oil some at a time, stirring to coat with oil. Stir fry until the bean curd starts off evolved to brown, 6-8 mins. Upload numerous beneficiant dashes of liquid smoke while stirring.

Upload the zucchini, snow peas, toddler corn and bell pepper to the sauté pan or wok. Stir in the broccoli florets and darkish green scallion tops, then stir-fry until the florets start to show dark green, about two mins.

Drain and rinse the bean threads. In a huge serving bowl, toss the bean threads and stir-fry mixture collectively. Serve right away.

Hot Garbanzo Beans with Sun Dried

That is a great go-to party dip for adults and children. Serve it with Baked Pita Chips or clean greens like jicama or celery. You could even spread it on a chook sandwich.

Ingredients

Tomatoes 2 tbsp olive oil

Four solar-dried tomatoes, thinly sliced two garlic cloves, thinly sliced

Half of the medium onion, thinly sliced

Half to 1 dried New Mexico pepper, stemmed and overwhelmed (or 1 tsp dried purple pepper flakes (or to flavor))

1 (16oz) of can garbanzo beans water

Salt and ground black pepper

Ingredients

Warm the oil in a small sauté pan over medium warmness. Add the solar-dried tomatoes, garlic onion, and New Mexico pepper and sauté until the onion begins to brown. Upload the garbanzo beans and retain to sauté for about five mins, or until the garbanzo beans start to brown. Upload enough water merely to cover the garbanzo beans then stir properly. Reduce heat and simmer for about five mins, or until the liquid is gone. Add salt and black pepper to taste and serve right now.

Masala Potatoes

Bombay Potatoes are chatpate masala also. Lined with spices and geared up in below 15 minutes, they double up as an appetizer and essential direction.

Ingredients

Three tbsp margarine

1 tbsp black mustard seeds

1 fresh long slim pink cayenne pepper, stemmed 1/2 tsp complete black peppercorns

Two medium onions, coarsely chopped one pink bell pepper, cored and diced one tsp turmeric

Half tsp floor coriander 1/2 tsp salt

1 to three tsp floor cayenne pepper

Four or 5 medium potatoes, unpeeled, parboiled and reduce into 1-inch chunks 1/4 cup of hot water

Juice of 1 lemon

Instructions

In a large pan, soften the margarine over medium warmth. Add the mustard seeds and sauté approximately two mins. Upload the whole cayenne pepper, peppercorns, onions and bell pepper and sauté around three mins, or until the onions are tender.

Add the turmeric, coriander, salt and ground cayenne. Stir properly into the mixture. Upload the potatoes, water, and lemon juice and stir nicely. Reduce the warmth to low and simmer, protected for three-five minutes or till the sauce thickens. Put off the entire cayenne pepper before serving.

MexiCorn

I merely made this dish. Scrumptious! I'm sorry about altering recipes. However, I handiest delivered it. I introduced a red bell pepper and a few dried basil, to taste. Changed into out of banana peppers, so I used chili flakes.

Ingredients

2 tbsp margarine

One small purple bell pepper, cored and coarsely chopped

One fresh inexperienced Anaheim pepper, stemmed and coarsely chopped one clean inexperienced jalapeno pepper, stemmed and coarsely chopped 1 (12oz) can complete kernel corn, drained

Salt and ground black pepper

Instructions

In a small saucepan, melt the margarine over medium heat. Combine the peppers into the pot and simmer for two-3 minutes. Add the corn and stir nicely. Low the heat, cover and simmer for 3 – five minutes, stirring regularly to prevent burning. Add season, salt and pepper all to taste and serve piping hot.

Hot Nutty Butternut

Butternut squash isn't only for dinner. At center Bar in new york metropolis, chef/owner Michael Lomonaco makes it right into a syrup for a butternut hot toddy.

Ingredients

Squash four tbsp margarine

One clean red serrano pepper stemmed and minced half cup cashews, coarsely chopped

1/2 cup currants

Half cup chunky peanut butter 1 tbsp unrefined sugar

1 butternut squash, halved lengthwise and seeded Preheat oven to 400F

Instructions

Melt the margarine in a small bowl over low warmth. Add the serrano pepper and cashews and sauté for two mins. Add peanut butter and stir until everything melt, then add the sugar. Stir nicely and remove from the heat.

Butternut squash has a hollow space at the blossom end and a protracted solid section that extends to the stem.

The use of a paring knife, make numerous 1/four-inch cuts in the flesh extending from the cavity to the stem give up. The area the squash halves in a baking dish and cover the cut surface with the nut combination. Divide the remaining nut combination among the two cavities. Bake for like 60 to 70 mins, or until a fork can be wick inserted through the skin into the stable phase of squash.

Spicy Hoppin' John

Historically, Hopping John is served inside the South at New yr's because the black-eyed peas represent cash—they're meant to usher in prosperity in the coming year. Our model, with all its veggies, is brisker. This side dish can be made in a day beforehand and is, in fact, higher after the flavors have had a hazard to meld.

Ingredients

6 scallions

tbsp extra virgin olive oil

One carrot peeled and thinly sliced one celery stalk, thinly sliced

One purple bell pepper cored and julienned

1 or extra fresh long narrow red cayenne peppers, diced

1 (10oz) package deal frozen black-eyed peas, thawed and rinsed (or a 15oz can rinse) 1 bay leaf

1/2 tsp of salt

1/2 tsp of black pepper 1 tbsp liquid smoke

1 tbsp chopped garlic

1 (12oz) bottle dark beer Cooked rice

Instructions

Trim scallions. Do away with the darkish new tops and set aside. Reduce the white and mild green sections into 1/four inch thick slices.

Warm the oil in a big sauté pan over medium warmness. Add the carrot and stir well to coat with oil. Add the white and mild inexperienced sections of the scallions and the celery, reduce heat to low and sauté for two mins. Add the bell and cayenne peppers and sauté for about three mins or until the carrot begins to brown. Upload the black-eyed peas and stir well. Sauté for 1 minute.

Upload the bay leaf, salt, black pepper, Liquid Smoke, garlic, and beer. Stir properly and bring to a boil. Lessen the heat and simmer, blanketed, for about 10 minutes, or till the liquid is sort of wholly absorbed – there needs to be about 1/3 cup sauce nonetheless.

Thinly slice the darkish green scallion tops even as the mixture simmers. Then stir in half the scallion vegetables. Ladle the Hoppin' John over a bed of cooked rice and sprinkle with last scallion vegetables.

Killer Curry

Brief and accessible veggie curry dish that is guilt free! You may be innovative with it as soon as you have got a simple concept down. I made a few final week and introduced some leftover diced up the beef roast. It rocked!

Ingredients

1 (19oz) can garbanzo beans, drained, liquid reserved 2 (10oz) programs frozen chopped spinach

Four tbsp margarine

Two clean, lengthy slender pink cayenne peppers, stemmed and minced one fresh pink jalapeno pepper, stemmed and minced

Seven garlic cloves, minced

Three medium onions, minced

Two carrots, peeled, halved lengthwise and reduce into half-inch slices 1/2 cup slivered almonds

Half cup golden raisins two tsp ground cumin

One tsp ground coriander one tsp turmeric

tbsp paprika

Two tsp salt

One tsp floor black pepper 1/four tsp ground ginger

1 cup water

One yellow bell pepper, cored and reduce into 1/2 inch squares 2/three cup coconut milk

cooked rice, warm

Instructions

In a heavy saucepan, combine the liquid from the garbanzo beans and the frozen spinach. Location over deep warmness, cowl and permit the spinach to thaw.

In a large sauté pan, melt the margarine over medium heat. Upload the new peppers, garlic, and onions and sauté for 1 minute. Add the carrots and sauté for 4-6 minutes or until the onions are golden brown.

Stir in the slivered almonds, golden raisins, and garbanzo beans and stir well. Sauté for 1 minute. Upload the cumin, coriander, turmeric, paprika and ground ginger. Stir well and sauté for 1 minute. Add the thawed spinach and garbanzo liquid and water to sauté pan, stir adequately and simmer for 10 minutes.

Upload the bell pepper and coconut milk to the sauté pan and stir well. Lessen heat to low and simmer, covered, for 30 minutes. Serve piping warm with rice.

Polka Pepper Pasta

That is my version of a recipe from hunts.com. the equal besides I exploit my home made the sauce and extra of the entirety, due to the fact the serving length they listing is never enough for my hungry bunch

Ingredients

1/2 cup margarine

Three fresh pink jalapeno peppers stemmed and thinly sliced seven garlic cloves

Two substantial candy onions, quartered and cut into thick slices

One medium head cabbage, quartered, cored and reduce into thick slices salt and pepper to flavor

1 lb skinny noodles

Instructions

Fetch water into a big pot and bring to a boil to cook the noodles. Soften the margarine in a heavy sauté pan over medium warmness. Add the jalapeno peppers, garlic, and onions. Upload the cabbage to the container is complete. You may no longer be able to suit all of the cabbage in the pan at the start. However, you could add greater because it cooks down. Sauté, often stirring, for 15 to 20 mins or till all the cabbage is smooth and distinct. Season with salt and black pepper to taste.

Prepare dinner noodles al dente, according to package deal instructions. Drain it well and transfer to a large serving bowl. Upload the cabbage and blend properly. Serve piping warm.

Loco Lo Mien

Ingredients

One ancho pepper stemmed, seeded and torn into small portions

dried New Mexico pepper, stemmed, seeded and torn into portions half of cup boiling water

2-inch length fresh ginger, peeled and julienned one broccoli stalk

1/4 cup extra-virgin olive oil

1 lb extra company bean curd, tired and reduce half of the inch cubes two carrots, peeled and cut into 1/4 inch slices

Six scallions

1 (8oz) can sliced water chestnuts, drained

1 (15oz) can infant corn, drained 1 cup sliced mushrooms

One small zucchini, quartered lengthwise can cut into 1/2 inch portions one red bell pepper, cored and julienned

1 cup snow peas, trimmed and cut into half of the inch pieces 2 tbsp chopped garlic

Half of cup light teriyaki sauce one tsp ground black pepper

1 (10oz) bundle Chinese noodles or 1 lb angel hair pasta

Instructions

Placed the ancho and New Mexico peppers in a small bowl and poured boiling water. The area the ginger on the pinnacle of the peppers and set aside to cool to room temperature.

Fill a large pot with water and produce to a boil to prepare dinner the noodles.

Get rid of the broccoli florets from the stalk. Damage or reduce the florets into chew length pieces and set apart. Trim any leaves or difficult dry components from the broccoli stalk. Reduce the stem into 1/4 inch slices.

Warm the olive oil in a large sautépan or wok over high heat. Upload the bean curd and sauté for eight-10 mins or till the bean curd begins to brown. Upload the broccoli stalks and carrots and sauté for 3 – five minutes or until carrots start to brown.

Even as carrots are sautéing, trim the scallions. Get rid of the darkish new tops and set apart. Reduce the white and light inexperienced sections into 1/4 inch slices.

Add the white and mild inexperienced scallions, water chestnuts, infant corn, mushrooms, zucchini, bell pepper and snow peas to the pan and sauté it for three-five minutes. Upload the broccoli florets and sauté for two-three mins or until the florets turn darkish green but are nonetheless crispy.

Inside a blender or food processor, add the re-hydrated peppers, ginger, garlic, teriyaki sauce, and black pepper. Puree for 1 minute or until smooth.

Upload the purée to the greens and stir nicely. Lessen the warmth to low and simmer, blanketed, while you put together the noodles.

Prepare dinner the noodles al dente in keeping with package commands. While the noodles still on the heat, thinly slice the dark inexperienced scallion tops.

Drain noodles nicely and toss with the greens. Serve right away, with the dark inexperienced scallion tops sprinkled on top.

Red Hot Red Pepper Salsa

This salsa is my entire right now. I could eat all of it day long. Nearly every single factor on this smoky, highly spiced eating place fashion salsa spends some time on the grill. It makes me pretty. Due to the fact you understand how obsessed I'm with my rack (trace: genuinely obsessed). I started out off wondering I would merely grill the tomatoes and the pink pepper. Then I only type "went for it" and threw the entirety else on – the onion, limes, jalapeños or even the garlic.

Ingredients

1 tbsp greater virgin olive oil

1 or more sparkling lengthy slender pink cayenne peppers, stemmed and minced one medium onion, coarsely chopped

One pink bell pepper, cored and diced (or use 1 cup diced roasted bell pepper) 1/2 tsp ground black pepper

1/2 tsp salt 1 cup water

Instructions

Heat the oil in a small sauté pan over medium warmth. Add the cayenne peppers, onion and bell pepper and sauté for 2-three minutes or until the onion is visible. Upload the black pepper, salt, and water and decrease the heat to low. Cowl and simmer for 10 minutes.

Puree in a blender or food processor geared up with a chopping blade for 30 seconds to 1 minute, until no large portions of pepper stay. Serve warm.

About the Author

Joe Beam is author of several cookbooks on Vegan diet. He has written research papers on the topic and currently lives in California.

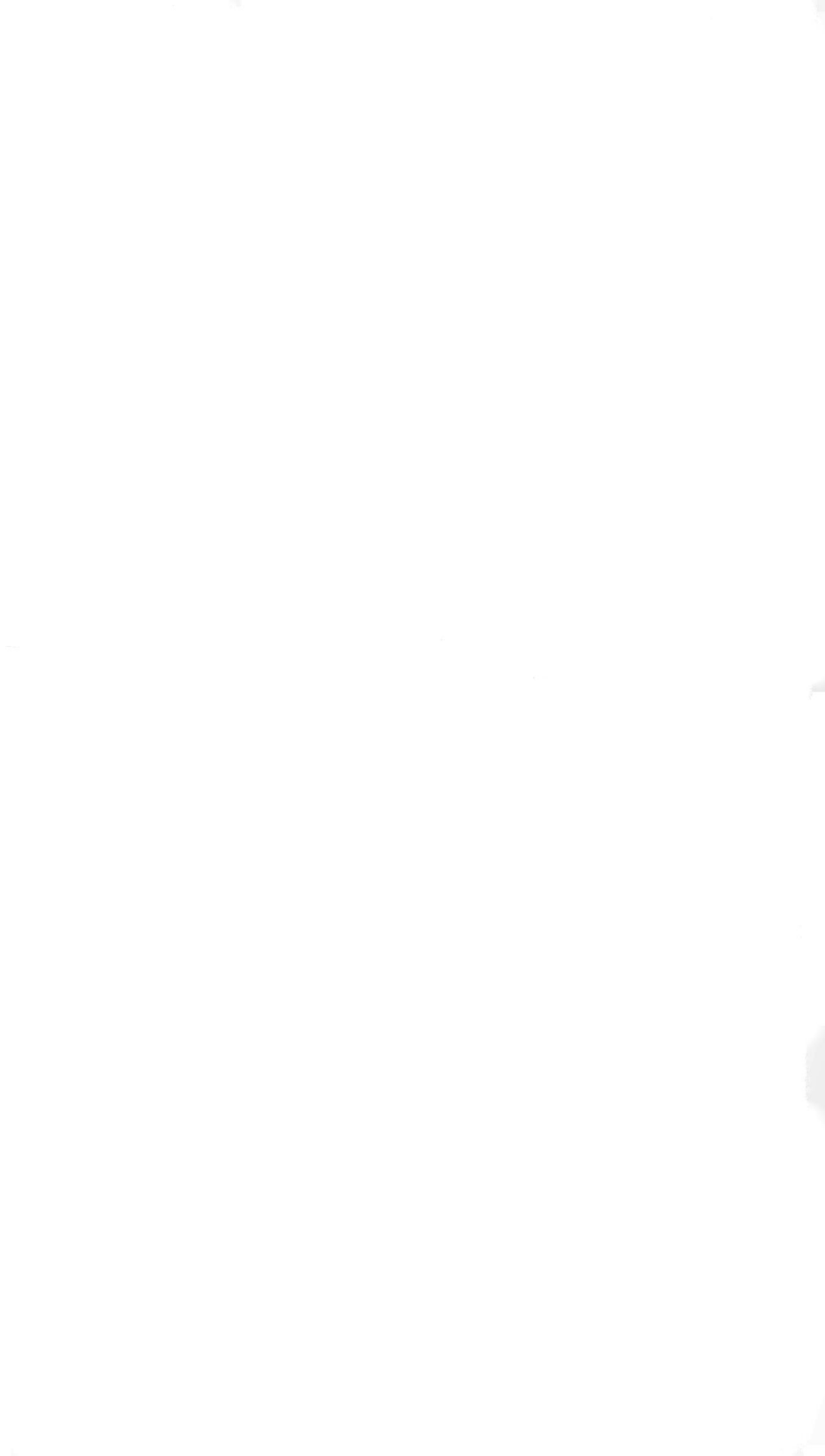

CPSIA information can be obtained
at www.ICGtesting.com
Printed in the USA
LVHW080843220222
711618LV00013B/693